The Power of the Mind to Heal

BOOKS, AUDIOS, AND MORE BY THE BORYSENKOS

BY JOAN BORYSENKO:
- *Minding the Body, Mending the Mind* (basic meditation and psychological healing practices), Bantam Books, 1987.
- *Guilt Is the Teacher, Love Is the Lesson* (healing the wounds of childhood and orienting to the Spiritual Self), Warner Books, 1990.
- *On Wings of Light: Meditations for Awakening to the Source*, co-created with artist Joan Drescher, Warner Books, 1992 (magnificent illustrations and meditations for humans from 6 to 106). There is also an audiocassette version of *On Wings of Light*, narrated by Joan, with an original soundtrack produced by Gordon Burnham and Jim Richards.
- *Fire in the Soul: A New Psychology of Spiritual Optimism*, Warner Books, 1993.
- *Pocketful of Miracles: A Book of Daily Spiritual Practice*, Warner Books, 1994.

Hay House, Inc. Audiocassette Series by Joan:
- Meditations for Relaxation and Stress Reduction
- Meditations for Self-Healing and Inner Power
- Meditations for Healing the Inner Child and Improving Relationships (for women)
- Lecture and Meditation on: Invocation of the Angels and Lovingkindness
- Lecture and Meditation on Overcoming Depression
- Lecture and Meditation on Forgiveness and Compassion
- Minding the Body, Mending the Mind. Joan reads her classic *New York Times* bestseller, a four-tape set.

Also from Hay House, Inc.:
- *Inner Radiance* Engagement Calendar. This calendar features inspiring reminders from Joan, and magnificent healing art mandalas created by Miroslav (Miron) Borysenko.

Other Audiocassettes by Joan and Miron:
- *The Power of the Mind to Heal*, Nightingale-Conant, 1993. Six double-sided cassettes that provide up-to-date medical and psychological knowledge about healing, enhanced by wisdom from the world's great spiritual traditions. The set includes several guided meditations and a set of inspiring prayer cards.
- *Workshops and lectures* by Joan and Miron on different aspects of mind/body healing, meditation, spiritual optimism, psychological healing, and prayer.

Videocassette by Joan Borysenko
- *An Evening with Joan Borysenko* is a 60-minute video of one of Joan's inspirational talks produced by Hartley Films.

To order books, tapes, music, the *Circle of Healing* newsletter, to find out about our teaching schedule, or to inquire about sponsoring a program in your area, please write or call: MIND/BODY HEALTH SCIENCES, INC., 393 Dixon Road, Boulder, CO 80302-7177 (303) 440-8460 — phone, (303) 440-7580 — fax

The Power
of the Mind
to Heal

Joan Borysenko, Ph.D., and
Miroslav Borysenko, Ph.D.

Hay House, Inc.
Carlsbad, CA

Published and distributed in the United States by:

Hay House, Inc., P.O. Box 5100, Carson, CA 92018-5100

Edited by: Jill Kramer
Designed by: Christy Allison

Library of Congress Cataloging-in-Publication Data

Borysenko, Joan
    The power of the mind to heal / Joan Borysenko and
Miroslav Borysenko.
       p.   cm.
    Includes bibliographical references.
    ISBN 1-56170-144-0 : $12.00
    1. Mental healing. 2. Mind and body. 3. Medicine, Psychosomatic.
I. Borysenko, Miroslav. II. Title.
RZ401.B7325 1994
615.8'52–dc20   94-31668
                                                  CIP

ISBN 1-56170-144-0

00 99 98 97 96   7 6 5 4 3
First Printing Hardcover Edition, October 1994
Second Printing (First Tradepaper Edition), September 1995
Third Printing, January 1996

Printed in the United States of America

This book is dedicated to the ones we love.

Contents

Contents

Acknowledgments

We hold this manuscript in heart and hand and give profound thanks to one another for the patience to stay in a relationship for 23 years. Early in our marriage, a spiritual teacher, Reverend Chris Williamson, reminded us that those who wish to make quick spiritual progress don't retire to monasteries, they get into relationships! We thank each other for what we have learned about love, and thus about healing, through the commitment we have made to one another and to our children.

Thanks to Georgene Cevasco of the Nightingale-Conant company, Joan's producer for the audiocassette program *The Power of the Mind to Heal*, which was the seed from which this book flowered.

Thanks to those who mentored us. Miroslav (Miron) wishes to thank the late Professor William Hildemann, who taught self-respect and kindness, as well as immunology. Other mentors have been Herbert Benson, M.D., who provided the space and interest for both our research in psychoneuroimmunology and Joan's clinical training in behavioral medicine; Jon Kabat-Zinn, Ph.D., whose Relaxation and Stress Reduction Clinic at the University of Massachusetts Medical Center was an inspiration and early model for the Mind/Body Clinic that Joan co-founded with Drs. Ilan Kutz and Herbert Benson; Stephen Maurer, M.A., who added so much to both the Mind/Body program and to my life; David McClelland, Ph.D., whose lively mind was always thinking up the next experiment; Robin Casarjian, M.A., whose teachings on love and forgiveness have been a personal as well as a professional blessing to us both; Rick Ingrasci, M.D., who taught us the power of community healing circles; Sogyal Rinpoche, who re-inspired our meditation practice; Elizabeth Lawrence, M.A., whose Mari-El healing work was very instructive and of great help; Joan Drescher, who taught us so much about beauty and healing; and Rachel Naomi Remen, who has always been both an inspiration and a friend. Our work is very broad-based and synthetic, resting on the shoulders of other colleagues too numerous to mention here. Either you have been cited in the text or you know who you are. Thank you for providing the scaffolding on which we have been privileged to build.

A super-special thanks to our dear friends and colleagues, Barbara Dossey, R.N., and Larry Dossey, M.D. Sometimes we think there is only one of us, occupying four bodies. Larry's work has been an enormous influence and framework for our thinking. Surely he has one of the brightest minds and warmest hearts of our times. Barbie's work on ritual and healing is also exceptional, as is their loving relationship, which continues to inspire our own.

Thanks, too, for the support of the friends who have shared our interest in mind/healing and spiritual growth, taught us new things, and loved us both individually and as a couple: Celia Thaxter Hubbard (a.k.a. Mother Goose), Peggy Taylor, Alan Shackelford, Ursula Reich-Henbest, Loretta and Bob LaRoche, Olivia Hoblitzelle, Roger Paine, Rima Lurie, Kristi Jorde, Rodrigo Rocha, Carolina Clarke, and Renee Summers.

Our children, too, have been wonderful teachers and great friends. Thank you Natalia, Justin, and Andrei. Living in an extended family with Natalia, her husband Shawn Harvey, and their son (yes, we're grandparents!) Aleksandr has brought the psychological construct of "social support" to a very real level. We should all be so fortunate.

We wish to express our deepest gratitude to the people we have been privileged to work with over the years, Joan's clients, and the participants in our workshops. We have learned a great deal from many of you. The stories of clients and friends whose names appear in quotation marks have been changed to protect their anonymity, as have any identifying aspects of their stories. At times, the stories of several people have been combined into a representative composite.

And finally, thanks to Louise Hay and all the wonderful people at Hay House who have been such strong supporters of our work. Without the kindness and commitment of Reid Tracy, in particular, this book would not have come into being.

Introduction:
The Healing Present

One late September morning in 1986, I was preparing to facilitate a session in the mind/body clinical program that I had co-founded and was director of at Boston's Beth Israel Hospital. The group consisted of about 20 participants. Some people who attended had cancer, a few were HIV positive, and most had an array of chronic or stress-related illnesses that ranged from high blood pressure to migraine headache to serious environmental sensitivity. I arrived in our sunny, spacious group room armed with an economy-sized box of tissues, having contracted our kids' back-to-school cold.

As I took my seat among the circle of chairs, sniffing and snorting, 40 eyes stared at me with dismay and outright disbelief. I could practically hear the thoughts: *My God, she meditates, she's stress-hardy, she eats a low-fat diet with lots of fruits and vegetables, and she's sick!* I felt a little bit like the Pope, caught walking out of a brothel. I couldn't help thinking of how different the response would have been had the group consisted of people interested in anthroposophic medicine—a form of natural healing that grew out of the work of the German physician, Rudolf Steiner. Anthroposophic physicians would have been delighted by my cold, even more so had I been running a fever, because they believe that such minor illnesses stimulate the immune system and help prevent chronic, autoimmune diseases such as arthritis or lupus.

The fact is that we don't really understand the health value of having a cold, or all the variables that predispose us to get one. But my patients' shocked, disappointed response upon discovering that I was human and perfectly capable of getting sick was great grist for the mill of our mutual learning and discovery. It reminded me of the response of the old testament character Job's three friends to his anguished question, "Why me?" after his children had been killed, his fortune decimated, and his health taken away. The three scared friends concluded that Job must have done something wrong, that he must have offended God, because otherwise bad things didn't happen to good people. The reasoning behind their attitude was that if we're really, really good and do everything just right, bad things won't happen. It's an interesting quirk of human nature that most people would prefer to experience guilt rather than the feelings of helplessness associated with not knowing why we've fallen ill.

In this book, we'll consider the intriguing questions of why we get ill and how we can participate in our healing. The day that I ran the mind/body group while alternately sneezing and blowing my nose, the participants and I had a wonderful discussion about the difference between curing and healing—a crucial difference that we will explore together in the pages to come. At the most basic level, *to cure* means to restore to health. When we are ill, naturally, cure is among our most fervent desires. As a former cancer cell biologist with a doctorate in medical sciences from Harvard Medical School, I know a lot about the pathways through which the body gets sick and how it recovers. I also know that *there is no such thing as an incurable illness.* Even when people have widely metastatic (traveling from one site in the body to another) cancer or AIDS, there are a few well-validated reports of complete cure. Researchers hope that by studying the few people who have "spontaneous remissions," we may be able to learn important principles that will help others as well.

I put the term *spontaneous remissions* in quotations above because if you ask people who have had remissions to tell you how their recovery came about, they rarely use the word *spontaneous.* In contrast, most will usually relate a story characterized by hard work—that is, a sincere effort on their part to modify physical habits, to find the right physician or treatment, to heal emotional wounds, to forgive themselves and others, or to find deep spiritual meaning in life. Many such people will tell you that the illness was a catalyst for their healing, and that even if a "cure" hadn't been the end result, their enriched experience of life would have made the illness worthwhile.

In the chapters that follow, you will read about the fascinating scientific breakthroughs in mind/body medicine that teach us how healing can sometimes lead to physical cure. But you will also read the stories of people who healed their lives, even in the process of dying. I used to joke with my patients that if they were using mind/body techniques to live forever, they were going to be very disappointed. As that great American philosopher Redd Foxx once said, "All those health food nuts are going to feel mighty foolish when they're lying there in the hospital dying of nothing." Our time on this earth, in these bodies, comes to a natural end when our "lifestory" is complete.

Naturally, it's important to take responsibility for our physical health—through exercise, proper nutrition, and the body/mind approach, but healing is really much less about the quantity of our lives than the quality.

Take a minute and think about your answers to the following questions, and make sure to be honest with yourself:

Do you get up in the morning with a feeling of joy and excitement about the new day, or, on the other hand, are you often depressed or anxious?

Do you feel a sense of confidence and inner peace, or are your moods determined by what other people think of you?

Do you live your life in the moment, with a feeling of gratitude and connectedness to the world, or do you live mostly in mental movies about the past and the future?

Do you feel the breeze and see the clouds and leaves when you walk outside, or are you too busy thinking about your income taxes or something you could have said or done differently?

> *Is your* heart open? Do you tend to see
> the best in yourself and in other peo-
> ple, or is it clogged with judgments?

Remember John Lennon's old line, "Life is what is happening when you're making other plans"? The best measure of a full life is not in its length, but in its love. When philosopher and writer Aldous Huxley was dying, he was asked, in light of the great knowledge he had accumulated, what, if anything, he would have done differently. His response was, "I would have been a little kinder." Kindness and compassion are, indeed, the heart of healing. It is a splendid confirmation of heart-knowledge that scientific studies indicate that love truly is the healer. The heart, the immune system, the hormones—they all respond in a positive way to the flow of compassion and connectedness we have to ourselves, to others, to nature, and to a larger Whole.

My role model for the *compleat* healer is a 12th-century Christian mystic, a Benedictine nun by the name of Hildegard of Bingen. Hildegard was the premier physician of her day, a pharmacologist with a wealth of knowledge about the herbs from which most of our modern-day pharmacopoeia was derived. She also described the circulation of the blood well before English physician Sir William Harvey did, although the discovery is usually attributed to him. Furthermore, Hildegard was a mystic who had many divine visions, during which she often heard the celestial music that people sometimes hear during near-death experiences.

An excellent composer, Hildegard transcribed this music, much of which is available today. My favorite cassette of her compositions is called *A Feather on the Breath of God*. Listening to her music, I feel a shift in my emotional energy—one that is no doubt accompanied by an outpouring of small proteins called neuropeptides—which send a message of peace and well-being throughout my body. Hildegard also had the artistic sisters in her convent paint her visions, many of which are sacred circles, or *mandalas*. While gazing at her art, one can also feel a shift to a deeper level of peace, a place where we feel a connectedness with the vastness of possibility that we may call God or Universe.

Hildegard believed that a complete understanding of healing had three parts. First, she said, we need science. I wholeheartedly agree. Prayer, emotional healing, and spiritual awakening are all a part of healing, but they in no way displace the proper role of science and medicine. The second aspect of healing is what Hildegard called a healthy mysticism—that which inspires us to wholeness. It is my hope that the stories of healings you will read about in these pages will not only present you with a healthy mysticism, but also inspire you spiritually. Hildegard's third aspect of healing was the use of art, for although science and mysticism lay the foundation for healing, she believed that it is the artist's special role to be the awakener of the people.

What did Hildegard mean by awakening? She believed that each of us carries our destiny inside us like a seed, and that as we encourage that seed to grow, we come into our fullness as co-creators of the Universe. The joy of creativity, and what Hildegard called "the awakening of the heart from its ancient sleep," is what we might think of as being fully alive. All of us have experienced moments of aliveness, often those times when we find ourselves fully present in the moment rather than being lost in fears about the past or worries about the future.

One New Year's Day when our grandson Aleksandr was about seven months old, we were taking down the Christmas tree. I was unstringing a length of gold stars, and as I crossed the room to give them to him, his entire body began to shake with excitement. That's being fully alive! His excitement was contagious, and I found myself in one of those timeless moments where colors seem brighter than usual, as if a thin veil has fallen away and revealed the true splendor of the world. I felt a sense of union with myself, with Alexsandr, and with the larger Whole. These moments of wholeness, or holy moments, are also healing moments when we exit the limiting cocoon of the stories we usually tell ourselves about life and enter into the sphere of unlimited possibility.

Holy moments are doorways where *chronos*—linear clock time, meets *kairos*—eternal timelessness. I believe that these are the moments when curing can sometimes occur—both through physical pathways, and through a grace that transcends the physical. For example, every so often I hear about a healing that defies medical science. Among the more than 60 "spontaneous remissions" that were meticulously documented at the shrine of the Virgin Mary at Lourdes, there is a case of a woman, blind since birth as the result of a shriveled optic nerve, who could suddenly see. Now, standard medical training tells me that a shriveled nerve cannot regenerate, yet it must have. At our current level of knowledge, we would have to call this a miracle. Perhaps in the future we will discover physical pathways for such instantaneous healings. For now, I attribute them to the power of faith to bring us into a healing moment where the two worlds touch.

Much of the research and insights in this book are the combined work of my husband Miroslav (Miron) Borysenko and myself. So far, I've been talking to you (Joan, that is), but at other times I'll be speaking for us both, replacing the "I" with "we." Even when I seem to be expressing sentiments that are exclusively from my own experience, Miron is a silent partner. He's been there, by my side, for nearly my entire adult life. Together we've made sense of our lifestories and found some of the wisdom in our wounds. Together we've healed and learned about healing. Let me introduce my partner and co-author Miron to you now.

Like me, Miron is a Ph.D., a medical scientist. We met and became a couple in 1971 when he was an assistant professor of anatomy and cellular biology at the Tufts University School of Medicine in Boston, and I was a graduate student at Harvard Medical School, just finishing my dissertation. After I finished my Ph.D. and a postdoctoral fellowship, I joined the Tufts medical faculty in 1973. Miron and I taught together at Tufts for almost a decade, pursuing independent research. My specialty was cancer, and Miron's was immunogenetics and then comparative immunology—a study of the evolution of the immune system.

In 1978 I returned to Harvard Medical School to complete a second postdoctoral fellowship in behavioral medicine. Since

Miron was eligible for a sabbatical, he took a visiting professorship at Harvard at the same time. Both of us became fascinated with the fledgling field called psychoneuroimmunology. For the first time, we shared a common research interest. I went on to finish my training in clinical psychology, and in 1981 (in collaboration with Herbert Benson, M.D., and Ilan Kutz, M.D.), I had the pleasure of co-founding the Mind/Body Clinic at Boston's Beth Israel Hospital that you've already been introduced to. That clinic grew out of Benson's pioneering work on the relaxation response (the integrated set of physical changes that accompany the meditative state); the work of Dr. Jon Kabat-Zinn, whose relaxation and stress disorders clinic at the University of Massachusetts Medical School in Worcester was an inspiration and early model for our own clinic; as well as Dr. Kutz's tremendous insight as a psychiatrist and my own long-term interest in yoga, meditation, cancer, and healing.

In 1987, Dr. Benson's Division of Behavioral Medicine, which was the home of the Mind/Body Clinic, moved to another of the Harvard teaching hospitals, the New England Deaconess. In that year, my first book, *Minding the Body, Mending the Mind,* which was based on our clinical program, was published. To our great surprise, it was a bestseller, probably because it is clear, accessible, and very practical. I still get grateful letters from people who learned how to meditate, to use creative imagination, and to begin the process of emotional and physical healing by working with that book. A year after its publication, I decided to leave Harvard for a variety of reasons—to make more time in my life for family and friends, to write more books, and to teach and travel. My growing interest in spirituality was also best pursued outside of the academic setting, although Miron and I have lectured at a large number of hospitals that are very receptive to the marriage of medicine, psychology, and spirituality.

In 1989, Miron left his tenured faculty position at Tufts Medical School, and together we founded a company called Mind/Body Health Sciences, Inc. Our vision is "healing society through healing the individual." We teach together in many settings—hospitals, retreat centers, places of worship, and a wide variety of civic organizations.

Over the years, I have written several other books: *Guilt Is the Teacher, Love Is the Lesson* takes a deeper look into the psycho-spiritual framework for healing. It is a book about transforming the wounds of childhood into wisdom and compassion so that we can begin to operate out of our Higher Self rather than our perceived limitations. *Fire in the Soul: A New Psychology of Spiritual Optimism*, is a book about the questions that arise in our hearts when we are diagnosed with serious illness or go through a crisis that puts us face to face with our most deeply held beliefs. Albert Einstein was once asked what the most important question was that a human being had to answer. He replied, "Is the Universe a friendly place or not?" *Fire in the Soul* is a companion to that question, and, I hope, a guide to finding spiritual optimism in the darkest nights of the soul.

During the time that I worked at the Beth Israel and New England Deaconess Hospitals, several people encouraged me to go over to Children's Hospital, where a remarkable healing mural graced the otherwise frightening and austere radiation therapy room. The artist, a woman by the name of Joan Drescher, had created a border of kites around the top of the room. The children lying on the radiation table could enjoy the kites, each of which contains a healing image from a different culture.

Without question, our body responds to the images that we create internally, and it also responds to the images that we see in our environment. When a leukemic child is told that he or she is to have a bone marrow test, it is often heard as a "bow and arrow test." Children have awesome, and sometimes terrifying, imaginations. Creating a healing environment where symbols of hope abound gives the child a positive message for their imagination that reassures them and that may even contribute to physical healing.

I was so impressed with Joan Drescher's work, and with the contribution of art and beauty to healing, that we co-created a book called *On Wings of Light: Meditations for Awakening to the Source*. Joan Drescher's painted images are deeply evocative, and the text leads the reader inward, to an experience of universal love.

My fifth book is called *Pocketful of Miracles*. It is a book of daily spiritual practices that is keyed to the energy of the changing seasons, the Great Medicine Wheel, and the four Archangels.

Drawing on the wisdom of a variety of spiritual traditions, from Tibetan Buddhism to Kabbalistic Judaism, from Sufism to Christianity, and from Native American teachings to Hinduism, the book is a structured series of short, daily practices and reminders for peaceful living.

In 1994, the Nightingale-Conant publishing company released an audiocassette series that I wrote and narrated entitled *The Power of the Mind to Heal*. It is the most comprehensive collection of both Miron's teachings and my own. It encompasses much of what I've covered in previous books as well as new material, tempered by the long years we have spent in this field and the remarkable experiences that we have had with people who were in the process of healing and also of dying. Hay House was very excited by the series and asked Miron and me to adapt it to book form. We are delighted to have been given this opportunity. In adapting the material, I've tried to keep some of the feeling of the tape series—the personal tone of a friend, or in this case, of two friends, speaking directly to you. In addition, the book covers significantly more ground than the tape series.

Miron and I share the belief that healing is really the simplest of matters. We are already whole. All we need to do is peel away the layers of fear that keep us out of touch with who we really are. The Buddhists have an image of the Higher or Spiritual Self as a sun that is perpetually shining even though the clouds of pain and illusion may temporarily hide it from view. Whether you call this sun the Inner Physician, your intuition, Essence, or Higher Self, our task as human beings is to discover and live from that place of wholeness. When we are in that place, we feel peaceful and spacious. The inevitable hurts and stresses of life are less taxing because we don't close down around them in fear. Rather, we stay more open to love and the infinite possibilities that are unfolding in every moment. We become a little kinder, a little lighter, and through our own healing we heal those who will come after us, and also those who have gone before. It's all a matter of remembering who we are and that when all is said and done, the entire awesome pageant of life is a drama about learning to love.

Joan and Miroslav Borysenko
Gold Hill, Colorado
Summer, 1994

PART ONE

Principles
of
Healing

CHAPTER ONE

THE POWER OF IMAGINATION

My interest in the body/mind connection and healing started simply enough at a Sunday dinner when I was about six years old. My Uncle Dick, who, as everybody knew, hated cheese, unknowingly ate two pieces of my mother's famous cheesecake, a mouth-watering confection smothered in strawberries and covered with a ruby-red glaze. About an hour after dinner, my mother commented to Uncle Dick that she was surprised that he had eaten the cake, knowing how much he hated cheese. At the mention of the word *cheese*, my uncle turned green and threw up all over the living room rug. At my tender age, this type of vivid demonstration left an indelible impression. Even though I didn't have the vocabulary to voice the obvious, it was clear that my uncle's stunning physiological reaction was not a biological effect of cheese. It was related, instead, to his perceptions about cheese, his mental images of what cheese represented.

From that moment on, I became an observer of the body/mind connection. For example, when we think an embarrassing thought—that is, when we replay embarrassing images on the movie screen of the mind, we blush instantly. As my friends and I reached adolescence, we blushed a great deal as "forbidden" images of the opposite sex flitted across our minds at the most inopportune moments. Blushing requires a veritable symphony of nervous system and circulatory system activity, yet the wisdom of our body does the bidding of our mind with no conscious prompting on our parts.

As a high school student, I became fascinated by the placebo effect (whereby an inactive substance or nonfoundational suggestion effects a particular occurrence). One winter day after lunch, a young woman became faint in French class. The teacher knew enough to have her lie down on the floor with her feet up while someone summoned the nurse. In the five minutes that it took for the nurse to arrive, a class member suggested that perhaps the girl's lightheaded condition was due to the pizza that many of us had consumed in the cafeteria for lunch. It had tasted a little bit different than usual, hadn't it? This suggestion precipitated a mini epidemic in my French class, as a number of students suddenly took sick. It is well known that suggestion has often been a precursor of epidemics, a phenomenon that is the dark side of the placebo effect.

In one fascinating study, a third of the women who got placebo chemotherapy treatments in a clinical trial testing the efficacy of the drug actually lost their hair! Another study—one that would never pass human studies committees today, I'm glad to say, involved pregnant women with such severe morning sickness that they had to be hospitalized. Half of them were given syrup of ipecac, a very potent drug that parents usually keep on hand to induce vomiting in case their children ingest poison. But these women were told that the ipecac would settle their stomachs. And for more than half of them it did—the power of their belief overriding the effects of this very potent drug!

As an intrepid teenage scientist, I wanted to know why and how we responded to the images in our minds, and which came first—changes in brain biochemistry that created new images—or new images that changed our brain chemistry. However, I can't pretend that my interest was entirely academic. When I was just ten years old, for no apparent reason, I fell prey to terrible mental images that I could not control. Nightmares of headhunters, poisonous snakes, and sudden death turned into "daymares." I went from being a normal, if slightly neurotic, fifth-grader, to being psychotic in a matter of days. Then, less than a week later, I also developed an explosive attack of obsessive-compulsive disorder, believing that the nightmare horrors would kill my family unless I performed a set of rituals that included almost nonstop handwashing, and reading things upside down, backwards, and three times without interruption. I finally had to leave school when I hallucinated headhunters in the corridor and flew into a terrified rage when my math teacher collected a test before I had the chance to erase each answer and rewrite it three times.

I had a stunning "spontaneous remission" from mental illness when an inner knowing told me that I had a choice. I could remain ill, or choose to recover through a tremendous act of will, promising myself that I would never perform another ritual. I am not implying that everyone with mental illness has a choice in the matter. But in retrospect, I believe that the illness and remission were specific gifts related to my life path in psychology and medicine. Falling into a state of hell certainly made me exquisitely curious about the events that had transpired. Where did the images come from? Could they have been triggered by the stress of moving to a new neighborhood and entering a new school? Were they the result of the nitrates from a few too many hot dogs clogging receptor sites for neurotransmitters? Were my brain cells affected by cosmic rays?

In college I studied psychology, biology, and philosophy and then went off to Harvard Medical School to study psychopharmacology—the interaction between drugs, the brain, and behavior. The summer before I started graduate studies at the medical school, I was hired to be the research technician for a cardiologist by the name of Herbert Benson, who was fascinated by the body/mind connection. He wanted to know if it was possible for monkeys to learn how to control their own blood pressure through biofeedback. While our ability to develop conscious control over some bodily functions may appear self-evident now, back in 1967 when I helped with that research, scientists believed that our autonomic nervous system (the division of the nervous system that regulates involuntary action) was entirely automatic. In other words, it functions by itself, without any possibility of conscious input.

The groundbreaking experiments of Benson and his colleagues showed that functions such as heart rate, blood pressure, and circulation could sometimes be brought under conscious control. Years later, that technology was honed and applied to people. For example, you can learn to abort migraine headaches by warming your hands; you can also learn how to raise and lower blood pressure. You can even alter your brain-wave state in ways that enable your mind to send clear commands, through vivid mental images, to your body.

The biofeedback research was interesting, but I turned out to be my own best laboratory for body/mind observation. The pressure of my studies, a failing marriage that had been entered into when my first husband and I were far too young, and the demands of early motherhood, put me over the top of the stress scale. And although you might think that a place for the training of healers would be nurturing, bringing out the best potential in the students, the atmosphere at Harvard in the late 1960s was downright toxic. We were trained to compete, to keep knowledge to ourselves, and to define success by how well we did on tests. All too often we were taught by humiliation rather than by encouragement, and a sense of bravado—almost a cowboy mentality—pervaded the air. Abuse of our bodies through hectic schedules, improper diets, and smoking cigarettes was the norm. And, while in those days nobody knew that social support—that is, time for loving and caring relationships—was the best protection against stress, our busy days and the endless competition left little time for building meaningful bonds with other people.

Certainly, medical school isn't the only toxic environment in which to work or learn. Many corporate settings embody the same principles: achieve, compete, win, and forget about any private life. *Stop and reflect for a moment.* What is *your* life like? Do you have time for yourself, time for relationships? If you work, what is the measure of success in your company? Is it consistent with your own ideas about success?

Studies of long-lived people (as opposed to those who die young) show that working more than 40 hours a week (particularly if your work isn't meaningful to you), experiencing loneliness on a regular basis, and getting less than eight hours of sleep on average correlate to rapid aging and premature death. Do your work life and home life reflect what means the most to you? Our dear friend, the humorist Loretta Laroche, quips that some of our tombstones might read, "Got everything done. Died anyway."

I'd never really thought about my definition of success, of what was most important to me, until I noticed the way that my body/mind reacted to the medical school environment. My insecurities and fears became glaringly apparent. I began to think that everyone else belonged at Harvard and that I was an impostor, that I must have gotten in by mistake. Did you ever think that if other people really knew you, if they could see into your soul, then maybe they would see just how unworthy you really were? Well, that's just how I felt—worthless, alienated, and lonely. Pretty soon my body began to respond to the pictures in my mind. I was always "awfulizing"—a wonderful word that the psychologist Albert Ellis coined. It means blowing things up out of proportion and creating mental movies of disaster—for example, parlaying a headache into a brain tumor and then worrying about how your family will ever survive without you.

Within about six months of starting graduate school, I got incredibly sick. Miron refers to my situation at that time as a medley of maladies. I developed high blood pressure and a cardiac arrhythmia, migraine headaches and a spastic colon, panic attacks and an anxiety disorder. And two decades before it was fashionable, I came down with a serious immune dysfunction. I had chronic bronchitis, repeat bouts of pneumonia, and even pleurisy. I'll never forget the moment that my doctor, who was obviously unaware of how a physician's words can become powerful hypnotic suggestions to a vulnerable patient, looked at me and shook his head sadly, commenting that he'd never seen the immune suppression syndrome I had except in homeless old men who'd lived for a long time in the streets. His comment, as scary as it was, was a wake-up call. I thought long and hard about the stresses of my comfortable and privileged life, and how my body was responding more to my attitude than to reality.

The fact that my doctors weren't much help was actually a blessing in disguise, as I couldn't get off the hook with a fast cure. Although my illnesses were well diagnosed, and abundant prescriptions were written, none of the doctors asked the most basic questions such as: *What is going on with you? What are your challenges? What gives you joy? What gives meaning to your life? How do you measure success?"* Had these questions been asked, the key to my healing might have been found. But in retrospect, I'm grateful for having been sick and for having been forced to figure out how to heal myself, because I learned so much in the process.

The road to my healing had two parts. The first part was simply learning to calm down the body/mind. This phase might be comparable to the joke about the holistic physician who counsels her patient to "take two meditations and call me in the morning." Although meditation can be just as powerful as a prescription medication, unless we probe the roots of our symptoms, meditation will simply mask our pain rather than helping us transform our trials into deeper levels of understanding and creativity. The second level of healing involved changing my negative perceptions about certain events in my life so that I could learn to experience things differently.

A lab partner in physiology who had been practicing meditation for years started me on both of these paths to healing. He had an easy, open way about him and rarely seemed stressed out by our professor, whom I secretly called "Der Fuhrer." One day I complained that our laboratory exercise was unnecessarily cruel. We were testing the amount of anesthesia necessary for a cat to tolerate various levels of pain. When finished, the graphs we constructed were supposed to match those in our texts. This, I fumed, was a pointless exercise. The research had already been done, and the graph was simple to understand. I refused to continue with the lab and was then humiliated in front of my peers as the professor berated me for being a squeamish woman, soft on animals, who ought to give up and go to nursing or veterinary school. Der Fuhrer gave me high blood pressure, or so I thought.

My friend "David" made it clear that although the professor might be wrong, I was giving him power by letting his behavior make me ill. I was the one in charge of my responses, not him. David used this episode to make a quick and penetrating diagnosis of how my mind worked in general. Anger and fear were driving my autonomic nervous system into high gear. I was living my life as if I were on the run from would-be persecutors who could pop up at any moment. This fearful imagining spawned a whole host of stress-related disorders. But, David counseled, there was a way to shift my physiology into a healing mode.

Anyone who meditates, he told me, is aware of obvious physiological changes brought about by the seemingly simple act of just focusing your mind in the moment. In that way, you quit living in the potent mental movies of disaster, regret, anger, and fear that not only rob your peace of mind, but can sometimes trick the body into believing that they are really happening. Once the mind is a little calmer, it is possible to develop much greater insight about your responses to life. My mother's advice was to count to ten before you reacted to someone in anger. If you do that, especially if you take ten belly breaths, you're likely to feel much more capable of responding creatively to the situation.

When you meditate, as we will practice later in the book, heart rate goes down, blood pressure drops, immune function improves, and there are a host of other beneficial changes that Dr. Herbert Benson went on to define as the relaxation response—the body's antidote to the fight-or-flight response. Within six months of learning to meditate, all of my symptoms disappeared. It seemed like a miracle at the time; yet, it was only the first step towards a deeper psychological and spiritual healing that continues today.

The Heart of the Matter

Sylvia and Sam had been married for 39 years. The last five were, in some ways, the best, like a well-aged wine. They were even sweeter than the early days of their marriage when Sylvia's blue eyes had twinkled with the secret that new life was growing in her womb. They had brought three beautiful children into the world, and four grandchildren. Life was good. Sam's leather business was flourishing. But somehow life had never seemed as precious until Sylvia was diagnosed with metastatic breast cancer. Every day after that, when Sam awakened, he would lift himself up on one elbow and look down at Sylvia. *Baruch Hashem*, Praise God, he'd utter in Hebrew. We have another day together. Five years after her diagnosis, Sylvia died at home, in their bed. Five months later, Sam had a heart attack and followed his beloved.

All of the old adages about dying of a broken heart, being heartsick, taking heart, and so on, are all based on fact. Many men, like Sam, become ill or die in greater numbers than would be statistically expected following the loss of their wives. Loneliness can truly be a heartbreaker. The sense of separation from life—whether through loss, depression, or protecting our vulnerability through angry cynicism can literally close down our hearts.

Heart disease is the number-one cause of death in the United States. Most of us are familiar with the risk factors—a diet high in saturated fat, high LDL cholesterol, obesity, lack of exercise, cigarette smoking, and diabetes, among others. But did you know that the majority of first heart attacks aren't related to any of these major risk factors? What do you think they *are* related to? Well, here's a hint. The majority of initial heart attacks occur on a Monday and are clustered between 8:00 and 9:00 A.M.! Some companies call this "parking lot syndrome." A Massachusetts study found that these Monday morning heart attacks were actually related to two key psychological factors: job dissatisfaction and lack of joy.

Our very dear friend, physician and writer Dr. Larry Dossey, sums up the attitude that predisposes one to parking lot syndrome in one telling phrase—"joyless striving." In his excellent book, *Meaning and Medicine*, Dossey speaks of joyless striving as the plight of the mythical figure Sisyphus, perpetually doomed to roll a rock up the hill, only to have it roll back down again.

The difference our attitude makes to the way we approach work is exemplified by an old story about three masons. They were all laying bricks when a man came up to them and asked each one what he was doing. The first one snapped, "I'm laying bricks. What the hell does it look like I'm doing?" The second one sighed, "I'm earning a living." But the third one gestured toward the sky and said, "I'm building a cathedral."

Pause and reflect on this story for a moment.... Now try on each of the attitudes that were depicted: angry cynicism, resignation, and inspiration. The best way to do this exercise is to close your eyes and relax yourself with a few deep breaths....Now, bring a memory to mind of a time when you felt angry cynicism. What was happening? Bring back as much detail as you can....Take a few letting-go breaths, and think of a time when you felt like the second mason—resigned to a joyless situation. Now once again, take a few letting-go breaths...and now think about a time when you really felt creative and inspired....Can you feel the difference in how your body responds to each of these attitudes?

Perhaps this exercise gave you an inkling of how physical response to our attitudes—which are really a pervasive set of images about life—might predispose us to heart disease. The feeling of joyless striving is a kind of resignation, a withdrawal from life, a turning-off of our very precious life-energy.

Did you feel a little tired, perhaps, when you remembered feeling resignation? Perhaps you felt your life energy surge once again, though, when you recalled a moment of inspiration and creativity. Life energy flows when we create, or when we help another person's creativity flower by encouraging them in some way. Think of the sense of joy and satisfaction that one can derive from the simple act of planting flowers, cooking a meal, writing a poem, solving a problem, painting a picture, dressing with flair, or doing your job to the best of your abilities. Creativity brings us to life, and by using our creativity we help bring the world into being.

While waiting for a plane in Buffalo, New York, recently, I met a young man who really brought creativity to his work. As the cashier at a news concession, he served a steady stream of travelers buying books or other small sundries. I was fifth in line, and feeling a little impatient. Then I heard his bright voice and noticed how "Bob" found something encouraging to say to each customer. He complimented one man on his choice of a book. A young mother's face glowed as he told her how clearly the baby in her arms was thriving from her love. By the time I was standing in front of Bob, I could hardly wait for my dose of what I call "lovingkindness." The measure of this man's success didn't lie in cashing out his register correctly at the end of the day or in bringing home a paycheck. It lay in how many individual human beings he'd been able to encourage and uplift.

Well, you might ask, what about people who work alone? How can they bring new life to their work? Barbara Dossey, an author, critical care nurse, and the partner of Larry Dossey, has a wonderful slide of a farmer alone in a field. He is bringing in a wheat crop with a harvester that cuts wide swaths through the waving fields of grain. The next slide is an aerial view of his work. The paths he has cut with his harvester have recreated Vincent van Gogh's famous painting of sunflowers! This attitude of playfulness goes hand in hand with creativity. It brings our hearts to life because we feel the inner wellspring of joy that is our birthright as human beings.

While it is often possible to approach our tasks in more life-affirming ways, there are also times when a work environment is so toxic that we are better off leaving. I have often lamented when patients or friends remained in job situations that seemed almost abusive, fearful that no better opportunity would come along. I've certainly done that myself at times. But I've been equally amazed at how a heart attack, a diagnosis of cancer, or in my case, a head-on collision, can suddenly shake us loose from these dead-end situations! When we wake up from the illusion that this lifetime lasts forever, a window of opportunity opens so that we can reassess priorities and make changes in our lives that are most consistent with living joyfully and lovingly.

Let's return to our three masons for a moment. While the joyless striver may be at increased risk for heart attack, the mason who responded with angry cynicism may fare no better. Cardiologist Redford Williams and his wife, therapist Virginia Williams, have written an excellent book, *Anger Kills*. Throughout many years of meticulous research at Duke University Medical School, Dr. Williams and his colleagues discovered that the toxic part of the

Type A syndrome isn't perfectionism, time pressure, or doing many things at once—it's an attitude of angry cynicism, hostility, and judgmentalness. *Think about your own attitudes for a minute.* Do you curse that jerk who cut you off in traffic? Do you tend to make sarcastic remarks? Is your head full of unkind judgments about strangers that you've never even met? Do you blow little things way out of proportion and look for that stupid so-and-so who is to blame?

Through many years of working with people with stress-related problems, chronic illness, cancer, and AIDS, I've come to believe that letting go of regrets, resentments, and the tendency to be critical is at the very heart of physical, emotional, and spiritual healing—not just from heart disease, but from *any* illness. The reason for this phenomenon is very simple. When we judge and criticize, we feel instantly separated from ourselves, from the ones we're blaming and from life itself. Our whole body contracts as our heart closes. The life-force just drains away. In the latter half of this book, we will be learning ways to let go of regrets and resentments so that we can open our hearts to the flow of universal love and energy that is always available to us.

Our friend and colleague Dr. Dean Ornish pioneered the first program for actually reversing atherosclerotic heart disease. His fine book, *Dr. Ornish's Program for Reversing Cardiovascular Disease*, is the only medically documented method of actually clearing the plaque out of blocked coronary vessels. Like all real healing methods, the program requires hard work. For example, there is both good and bad news in the area of diet. The bad news is that if you have heart disease and you follow the American Heart Association diet, you will continue to build up occlusive plaque in your arteries. A diet including animal products—even lean ones— is not consistent with reversing heart disease.

Dr. Ornish prescribes a very stringent vegetarian diet with no dairy products other than a little yogurt made from nonfat milk.

There is absolutely no added fat in this diet. Vegetables, for example, are sautéd in a little bouillon or water rather than oil. In addition to very moderate exercise, Dr. Ornish's heart patients learn to meditate and visualize their coronary vessels as clear and open. But just as important, patients work on opening their hearts to themselves and others. When we are able to love and respect ourselves, we project that love to others, and the quality of our relationships changes dramatically.

Dr. Ornish's program is really about making connections, about fostering our sense of belonging to the wholeness of life. Overcoming the separateness that many of us experience when we never feel quite good enough or lovable enough is a three-part process, according to Ornish: personal, interpersonal, and transpersonal. *At a personal level*, we have to heal the wounds of our past that keep us separate from ourselves. *At an interpersonal level*, once we have come to respect and love ourselves, then, and only then, are we capable of authentic intimacy with others. *At a transpersonal level* (that realm which encompasses the Wholeness that we may think of as God or nature), once we are comfortable in our own skins, we will be able to relate in a more meaningful way to that Great Mystery.

Many of the people we have interviewed about their near-death experiences report that feelings of connectedness were central to the event. While I have never been near death myself, I have had two empathetic, or shared, near-death experiences. When my mother was dying, both our son Justin (who was 20 at the time) and I spontaneously entered the light with her. As often as I'd heard other people's light experiences, I realize now that there are no words adequate to describe the kind of love that you experience. Perhaps the most deeply moving aspect for me was the sensation that I was completely known— mistakes and all—and that my soul was pure. This holds true for every person of good heart. Now, what is a good heart? It is nothing more than having the intention to live your life with as much kindness as possible, knowing that you'll still fall short of the mark many times.

When I opened my eyes after sharing the moment of my mother's death, the entire room seemed filled with light. It was as though all the atoms in the air, in the walls, in the bed, in the body of our son Justin, who was sitting directly across from me, were vibrating with life. When you are witness to magnificence of this sort, nothing is separate. Everything is connected with and interpenetrating everything else. As I looked over at Justin, he was weeping, and a look of pure joy suffused his delicate features. He looked like a blond, cherubic angel as he said to me, "Mom, the room is filled with light. Can you see it?"

When I nodded that I could, he whispered through his tears, "Grandma is holding open the door to eternity so that we can have a glimpse." Every so often we may get a peek into a realm so extraordinary that it communicates a reality far grander than any we could ever imagine. Our task, then, is to bring these glimpses down to earth and make them practical. Most people who have had near-death experiences summarize what they learned by saying that we are here, on this earth, where things seem separate from one another, precisely because these are the best circumstances in which to learn about love.

We like to think of *love* as a verb, rather than a noun. Love consists of words, thoughts, and actions that encourage the potential in ourselves and others. When we are gentle with ourselves, we create the space from which creative possibilities best emerge. And once we can encourage ourselves, we can also give this gift to others. And who, after all, is an "other"? During the "glimpse" I was given by my mother, it was obvious that seen from a slightly different level, there is only one being in the entire Universe, each of us like the facet of a single diamond.

When our youngest son Andrei was a junior in high school, he came upon Chief Seattle's famous speech imploring the white race to care for the land that the American government had just seized from the Native Americans of the Pacific Northwest. He called the rivers our brothers and reminded us that we are just one strand in the web of life. What we do to the web, we do to ourselves. Our love is shown through every action, not just toward other people, but to the earth upon which we live and to the animals that journey with us. When we choose to recycle our bottles, for example, we honor the connectedness of all things. When we choose to eat less beef because of the serious ecological damage that cattle ranching does, we also honor life.

Love is the basic teaching of every religion, no matter how some groups may have twisted that message out of fear or self-interest. The great first-century rabbi, Hillel, taught that the core of spiritual life was to "Love the Lord thy God with all thy heart, with all thy soul and with all thy mind, and to love thy neighbor as thyself." In practical terms, he said that that meant practicing the golden rule and treating others as you would have them treat you. This message is very familiar, of course, to Christians, as the true heart teaching of Jesus, who we may tend to forget, was also a first-century Jew. When the Dalai Lama was asked about the spiritual beliefs of Tibetan Buddhism, he replied similarly—and with great simplicity—that his religion was compassion.

CHAPTER THREE

THE HEALING POWER OF LOVE

We once saw a beautiful scene in a documentary about the life of Mother Teresa. She and several of her Sisters of Charity had appeared in Lebanon during the war, asking, "How can we help?" They were sent to a home for spastic children that was short-staffed. The children there seemed small for their ages, shrunken and stunted. They were suffering from an illness known as hospitalism, or failure to thrive, that often occurs in group homes for infants. Although the children are fed and changed, their needs are met on schedule with little chance for the give and take that is natural between infant and caretaker. The pituitary glands of these unloved children fail to put out enough growth hormone. In effect, the baby gives itself a die message since there is no one to receive it into life.

Mother Teresa was holding one such child in the palm of her hand. The baby's face was squeezed into what looked like a death mask, and its shriveled limbs were contorted in spasm. All she did was hold the baby and croon to it, looking at the child with great love. After a few moments, the baby began to smile, and its tortured limbs relaxed. When Mother Teresa was asked why she bothered to care for the sick and the dying since they had no hope of recovery, she replied that her job was simply to love them. That was enough.

Research indicates that love—what researchers often call "social support"—is critically important to staying well. In fact, social support is the best predictor of good health, more powerful than any health habit, including diet and exercise. There is a well-known study based on data collected about the health and lifestyles of 7,000 residents of Alameda County, California. Women who actually had many social contacts but reported feeling lonely (those who couldn't let the love in) had a 2.4 times greater risk of developing hormone-related cancers including uterine, breast, and ovarian cancer than those who felt connected. Women who actually did have fewer social contacts and also felt isolated had five times the risk of dying from these cancers!

As we'll discuss in the next chapter, our immune system is very sensitive to loneliness, providing a mechanism through which feeling unloved and isolated might actually affect our body's ability to reject tumor cells. Isolation also affects the metabolism of fat and cholesterol, predisposing one to heart disease. In a fascinating study that involved rabbits—whose cardiovascular systems are very close to those of human beings—cuddling and care actually protected the rabbits from most of the artery-clogging effects of a high-cholesterol diet. Delightfully, the findings were serendipitous. The laboratory technician who ran the study loved rabbits and patted them whenever possible. But since she was short, she could comfortably reach only about half of the cages. Incredibly, the rabbits she cuddled were protected from most of the harmful effects of the cholesterol.

Obviously, our diets are important, but they are not the entire determinant of our health. There is a small town in Pennsylvania called Roseto. About 30 years ago, epidemiologists decided to study Roseto because the level of heart disease there was very low. They expected to find a lean, bean sprout-munching group of marathon runners, but were they ever surprised to find that many of the residents were overweight, sedentary, cigarette-smoking carnivores. The health risk was high, so what was the explanation?

Well, it seems that the issue of social support accounted for the town's unusually good health. Rosetans were a particularly close-knit community, and their values had more to do with neighborliness and kindness than with materialism. Unfortunately, over the next 25 years, Rosetans became more like many of their fellow Americans. Acquiring things and keeping up with the Joneses became more important than spending time with family and friends. As this value shift occurred, the level of heart disease in Roseto rose to the national norm.

In 1945, about 85 percent of all Americans lived in extended-family situations. By 1989, only 3 percent of Americans lived in that fashion. During Miron's sabbatical year at the Beth Israel Hospital, he sometimes volunteered as a translator for new emigrants from the former Soviet Union who spoke Russian or Ukrainian. We became friends with a family that consisted of grandma and grandpa, their two daughters and their husbands, and their three grandchildren. Within a year of immigration, they had found a three-family house to share. We loved to have dinner with these folks because the long "table" was a patchwork of bridge tables, end tables, and old doors. At least 20 people were eating there at any one time. Other immigrants and newly made friends all showed up with something to add to the feast. Storytelling about the old country, as well as sharing the perils and challenges of their new life, created an atmosphere of intimacy and closeness. From a financial standpoint, these people were poor, but I realized that they were a lot wealthier than we were when it came to the commodity that counted most—love.

The 1967 Surgeon General's report on smoking and health tells a similar story. When age-adjusted death rates were compared for men who who were cigarette smokers versus those who were not, it turned out—as you might expect—that those who smoked had twice the death rate of those who did not. But when married smokers were compared to divorced nonsmokers, the death rate was about the same. Dr. James Lynch, who reported these statistics in his excellent book, *The Medical Consequences of Loneliness*, wrote that the person who compiled these statistics had quipped that if a man's wife was driving him to smoke, he had a delicate statistical decision to make!

The men who were most at risk for cigarette-related death were those who were single, widowed, or divorced. Why might this be the case? We might reasonably assume, for example, that married men eat more carrots or cantaloupe and thus are protected by higher levels of beta-carotene. But that was not true. The protective factor turned out to be marriage itself. Think back to Sam, the man we met at the beginning of the previous chapter who had a heart attack five months after his wife's death. There is a significant increase in illness and death for men who lose their spouses. Interestingly enough, this is not true for women. When Miron and I teach together, he often jokes that the reason for this discrepancy is that men are more invested in their relationships! But there's a more obvious explanation. *Stop and reflect for a moment. What could it be?*

Well, it seems that women, in general, tend to form social networks and have a variety of friends with whom they can share feelings and on whom they can depend. American men, in contrast, often have fewer friends—a more limited network for social support. Oftentimes, a man's wife is his best friend, and sometimes she is the only one with whom he can really share his feelings. So when a woman's husband dies, she has other people to support her emotionally. But when a man's wife dies, he's often lost his best or only friend and is much more likely to either *become* or *feel* lonely and isolated.

Dr. David Spiegel is a Stanford psychiatrist who has been running support groups for women with metastic breast cancer for many years. He observed that the support that women gave one another in these groups, coupled with instruction in how to cope with the illness, helped to reduce anxiety and depression. He admits, however, that he was very skeptical that these positive changes in the quality of life might have anything to do with how long the women survived. But when he analyzed data from a group of 36 women who had come weekly to the group for one year, in contrast to 50 women with the same illness and treatment who had not come to the group, he was surprised. Those who were in the support group, on average, lived twice as long as those who were not. Eight years after they had entered the group with cancer that was already metastatic, four of the women in the support group were still alive. Two subsequently died of causes other than cancer, but at the ten-year mark, two were still alive without recurrence!

Dr. Spiegel's research was featured on Bill Moyers' acclaimed Public Television series, *Healing and the Mind*. The dynamics of the group were actually hard to watch. Many of the women seemed depressed at the prospect of the losses they were facing, including the loss of their lives. Spiegel helped the women air their feelings, face the worst, and then learn to cope.

Too often, however, support groups are well-meaning but don't allow the real sharing of feelings that is so important to healing. I counsel people to avoid the kind of support group where feelings of fear or depression are seen as signs of failure. "Positive thinking" can sometimes amount to pushing away the very pain and fear that can motivate us to heal our lives. Pasting on a smile and repressing our fears so that they can work on us in an underground fashion is a tactic that is likely to create chronic stress and a far worse medical outcome. On the other side of the spectrum, however, some support groups help their members air their concerns, but then leave the partipants to marinate in their distress.

Once we've faced our fears, the most important thing is to learn how to live our lives—not only in spite of them—but in a fuller, more present way because of them. Fear can be a wonderful teacher of love.

CHAPTER FOUR

PSYCHONEUROIMMUNOLOGY:
Where Mind and Body Meet

In 1978, Miron took a year's sabbatical as a visiting professor at Harvard Medical School to begin doing research in a fledgling field called psychoneuroimmunology. Partway through the year, he returned to Tufts Medical School to attend a staff meeting for faculty who were planning the following year's immunology course. When he explained that the study of psychoneuroimmunology sought to establish a link between our thoughts and the function of our immune cells, he was met by a stunned silence. On the way out the door, one of his colleagues stopped him, literally pointing the finger of disbelief. "Do you really mean that you actually believe that what we think can affect the activity of lymphocytes?" he challenged.

Miron held his ground. He did believe exactly that, and research has backed him up. There is an old metaphysical principle stating that "thoughts are things." Now, that might be a workable concept for metaphysicians, but many conventional physicians still blanch at the concept. As Miron tells the story, within a few weeks of his announcing his new research interest, there was a joke afoot in the corridors that he had become a psychotic, neurotic immunologist!

Only a few years later, the fact that conditions such as stress have a serious impact on immunity is no longer in question. Temporary stress, like studying for an exam, can completely wipe out the body's interferon levels, literally reducing them to zero. Interferon is necessary for certain cells of the immune system to do their jobs. For example, one kind of immune cell is a lymphocyte known as the natural killer cell. Natural killer cells have two functions. First, they patrol the body and seek out virus-infected cells for elimination. Second, they seek out and destroy cancer cells. Unfortunately, current medical science has not yet found a cure for viruses, and cancer treatment is still in a very rudimentary stage. How incredible that our bodies have lymphocytes that can perform these important functions.

In students, the stress of exam week often results in colds, cold sores, or other "minor" illnesses—perhaps as a result of the poor natural killer cell activity brought about by low interferon levels. Have you ever gone through a particularly stressful period and then, right after it was over, contracted a cold or the flu? Probably so, but fortunately, the body recovers very quickly from acute stress and the immune dysfunction that accompanies it. In terms of our long-term health, chronic stress is much more important than short-term stress.

Harvard physiologist Walter Cannon first described the body's response to acute stress, which he called the "fight-or-flight response," in 1929. From time to time you may have opened your morning paper and found a photograph that defies belief—for example, a 110-pound mother lifting a two-ton truck off her injured child. These seemingly miraculous feats are due to a physiological symphony that plays flawlessly when we are faced with an emergency. Adrenaline pours out of the adrenal glands, causing blood pressure to rise and the heart to beat more forcefully. At the same time, sugar is liberated from storage in the liver and pours into the bloodstream. This rapidly burning fuel is quickly delivered to our muscles, giving us uncommon strength. Adrenaline simultaneously improves visual acuity, short-term memory, and mental sharpness. We can make decisions fast and then act on them. We can survive.

The fight-or-flight response is mediated by the sympathetic, or activating branch, of the autonomic nervous system. These neural pathways respond to fear by triggering an outpouring of adrenaline that is then broken down very quickly by the body. If you have a scare in traffic, for example, your body responds instantly. A minute later, calm prevails again unless you decide to wallow in anger or frustration. And often, that's exactly what we do. For example, sometimes the stress of marriage is so taxing that we finally get a divorce, but by hanging on to ancient anger for years, we turn an old situation into a current stressor. Stress then becomes chronic.

In 1936, physician and physiologist Dr. Hans Selye described the physiology of chronic stress, which he called the *general adaptation syndrome*. When rats were chronically stressed, he noticed that their adrenal glands got very big and that their thymus glands—the source of T-lymphocytes—became very small. Although little was known about the immune system in the 1930s, it was obvious that chronic stress led to increased illness. What Selye was observing had a great deal to do with a hormone called corticosterone. In humans the analogous hormone is called cortisol. When we are chronically stressed, the hypothalamus of our brain secretes a hormone called ACTH, or adrenocorticotropin. This hormone then binds to cells in the outer cortex of the adrenal gland and causes them to manufacture and secrete cortisol. Over time, the gland gets bigger and bigger if it is constantly challenged with the need to make more cortisol. In the short run, cortisol is a repair hormone. But in the long run, it is an immunosuppressant. Cortisol not only prevents the formation of new immune cells, it also inhibits the activities of the ones already in our system.

Hans Selye himself had a spontaneous remission from an often rapidly lethal type of cancer called mesothelioma. When his physician informed him that he might have only a few months left to live, Selye decided to write his memoirs. As he was poring through old journals, his memory was jarred by several painful situations that had occurred in his past. One of them was the theft of his research findings by supposed mentors when he was still in medical school. He reasoned that he could either release the old hurt or belabor it. He decided to let it go and leave it out of his memoirs. He continued the retrospective of his life in that manner— that is, letting go of old hurts. When he returned for a check-up about a year later, his physician found that the cancer had disappeared! Was his remission related to his practice of forgiveness and the relief of chronic stress? We have no way of knowing the answer to that question definitively, but it's certainly a reasonable hypothesis.

Chronic stress not only takes the form of long-held regrets and resentments, it also shows up as feelings of hopelessness and helplessness when we feel that we have neither the skills nor the strength to cope with the challenges of life. The best definition of stress that Miron and I have found is "the perception of physical or emotional threat coupled with the perception that our responses are inadequate to cope." The key words here are *perception* and *coping*.

Miron often jokes that two people confronted with a large black dog may perceive the animal very differently. On the basis of past experience, one person may love dogs and be attracted to the animal; the other may fear dogs and be repelled. But if the dog were growling and foaming at the mouth, both people would be afraid. Then, coping skills would become important. A poor coper might freeze at the sight of the dog, and a good coper might hide behind the person who had frozen!

Whenever Miron tells that story, I am reminded of the two hikers who are set upon by a lion. One drops to the ground and puts on his sneakers, while the other berates him for thinking that he can outrun such a beast. The one donning his sneakers replies, "I don't have to outrun the lion; I just have to outrun you!"

People who are good copers are often referred to as *stress-hardy*. Psychologist Suzanne Kobasa has identified three attitudes that sustain such individuals during demanding times. These attitudes are called the three *C*'s: challenge, commitment, and control. A stress-hardy person sees change and crisis as a challenge rather than a threat. Even when they cannot control the outer situation, they realize that they always have control over their response to the things that are happening. There is a wise, old saying that relates to this phenomenon: Suffering is inevitable, but misery is optional.

Stress-hardy people who can endure the inevitable sufferings of life without becoming mired in misery are often able to thrive in hard times because they are committed to a set of values that puts crisis and difficulty into a positive frame of reference. For example, people who have to work very hard, but who are committed to their jobs because they believe that they are helping people, are less stressed than those who do not feel this type of commitment. The *meaning* that we ascribe to any stressful situation—be it a job, an illness, or the death of a loved one—makes a tremendous difference in our ability to cope. At times it can mean the difference between life and death.

Viktor Frankl, the renowned psychiatrist who wrote the beautiful and inspiring book, *Man's Search for Meaning,* is a survivor of the Nazi holocaust who was finally liberated from Auschwitz at the end of World War II. He observed that people who could find some meaning in their suffering often managed to hang on to the will to live, and if the Nazis didn't kill them first, they often survived until liberation. These were the good copers. He also wrote about how people who lost the will to live often died within hours from heart attacks, or simply succumbed to infection. Frankl was one of the first people to write about psychoneuroimmunology: "Those who know how close the connection is between the mind of a man—and his courage and hope or lack of them—and the state of immunity of his body will understand that the sudden loss of hope and courage can have a deadly effect."

The molecular mechanisms through which attitudes such as helplessness, hopelessness, and despair can impact the immune system have to do both with the autonomic nervous system and some tiny proteins called *neuropeptides*. Our brains are like pharmacies, compounding a wide range of drugs that affect both our moods and all of our biological systems, including the immune system. For example, when threatened with death—that is, if a sabertoothed tiger had you in its jaws—thanks to neuropeptides called *endorphins* and *encephalins,* you would feel somewhat peaceful, sleepy, and numb as you took your place in the food chain. Our brains also secrete valium and other natural tranquilizers, as well as dozens of other peptides related to the control and expression of emotion.

When you react to the very thought of your boss as if he were a saber-toothed tiger, your body secretes chemicals that prepare you to die, rather than helping you to live. The amazing thing is that these drugs are pumped out of the brain into the bloodstream and eventually bind to the surface of all the cells in your body, the way that a lock fits into a key. They then affect the function of all your cells. The area of the brain in which thought is transformed into emotional response is called the *limbic system*. Cells of the limbic system are particularly active in the manufacture and secretion of neuropeptides—a direct line of communication between emotions and the body.

For example, let's say that you've just had a joyful thought. Better still, bring a joyful thought to mind right now. Take a few letting-go breaths, close your eyes, and either recall something that made you happy, such as a baby's first smile or a delightful joke, or imagine something that might make you joyful in the future. Allow yourself to imagine—that is, to enter into—the scene with all your senses. What do you see or sense around you? Above and below you? Are there any sounds? Any special fragrances? Are you moving, touching, sitting, standing? What is the emotional, or deep-felt sense of the memory in your body? Now, if you've recalled joy, pause for another minute or two and really notice how your body responded to joy. Feel it in your cells.

Perhaps you feel somewhat different now than you did a few minutes ago. Your brief meditation on joy caused cells in your limbic system to release neuropeptides that crossed the blood/brain barrier and entered your bloodstream. In a matter of seconds, these clever little chemicals fit into receptor sites all over your body. When the key slid into the lock, various genes in your cells were turned on or off, starting or stopping the synthesis of proteins. Depending on what proteins were activated or deactivated, the function of all your systems was potentially altered. This is one of the many pathways through which thoughts become things.

So, if you feel joy, every cell in your body responds to that emotion. And if you are depressed, that image, too, is broadcast throughout the entire body/mind by the neuropeptide system. Furthermore, the brain is not the only organ that makes neuropeptides. The cells that line your gut are also neuropeptide factories, as are some lymphocytes. So what goes on in the digestive tract or the immune system in turn affects brain function and mood. Dr. Candace Pert, a neuroscientist who was one of the co-discoverers of the endorphins, has quipped that neuropeptides released by the gut may be the physiological basis of gut feelings!

Some of us are very aware of the way that our moods affect our bodies—how anxiety tenses the muscles, how depression leads to fatigue, how joy creates energy, and how gratitude and love open the heart. Dr. Pert and her colleague, neuroscientist Michael Ruff, believe that the mind and body cannot be separated—that each cell is imbued with mind. Our very cells are conscious, aware beings that communicate with each other, affecting our emotions and choices. When people speak of the body/mind connection, they are often referring to only one side of the equation—the effect of mind on body. But body also affects mind. What we eat, whether we are touched, how and whether we exercise, how we breathe— all these seemingly physical acts have a profound effect on our moods and on our ability to be clear-headed, loving, and creative.

CHAPTER FIVE

TRAINING THE IMMUNE SYSTEM

The immune system has also surprised scientists by its ability to learn. Dr. Robert Ader, one of the founders of the field of psychoneuroimmunology, discovered that the immune system can be trained in the very same way that Pavlov trained dogs to salivate at the sound of a bell. The dogs were given meat powder, which caused them to salivate. But if Pavlov paired the presentation of the meat powder with the ringing of the bell, soon the animals salivated to the sound of the bell alone. This is called *classical conditioning*.

Ader and his colleague, immunologist Nicholas Cohen, showed that if rats were given an immunosuppressive drug accompanied by apple juice, later on the rats would immunosuppress just by tasting the juice. Rats could also be exposed to drugs that enhanced different aspects of the immune system, and the immunoenhancement could be similarly trained.

Let's speculate on the possible implications of such conditioned learning. Perhaps a boss, an ex-spouse, or some situation is or has been a significant source of pain or chronic stress for you. When any cue associated with the situation comes up, your neuropeptides and autonomic nervous system go into a distress mode. The fact that it is easy to condition the immune system is a very practical reason to practice forgiveness so that we can leave old stresses in the past instead of reacting to them for a lifetime. In the same vein, since, as we shall see, feelings of joy and connectedness may enhance immune function, pictures of our loved ones, beautiful views, or forgiving thoughts may keep our immune system functioning optimally.

Miron and I had the great pleasure of working for several years with one of the most interesting psychologists of our time, Dr. David McClelland. McClelland, who spent most of his academic years as a professor of psychology at Harvard, is well known for his research on human motivation. Some people, he found, are highly motivated to achieve. If you present them with a set of pictures and ask them to write stories about what they see, you can get a spontaneous sample of their thinking—of the images in their minds. Such individuals have a lot of thoughts about solving problems, winning, coming out ahead, and getting things done. Other people are motivated by the need for power. These people write stories about dominating situations and other individuals, even though they may be in helping roles.

McClelland has done fascinating research linking the images that arise from our basic motivations, which are really our most deeply held values, and the function of our immune system. One of his most intriguing studies concerns the motive for unconditional love. When McClelland is trying to arouse thoughts related to a specific motive in a laboratory setting, he often uses films. A film about the Third Reich, for example, will generally increase power motivation. Finding a film that might bring out the love motive, however, has been a very challenging task.

Romantic love stories are a decidedly mixed bag. They may involve not only love, but also loss. And even if the love is uncomplicated in the movie, it might still tap into romantic problems in the viewer's own life. So, what's a researcher to do? McClelland settled on the idea of using a documentary on Mother Teresa. His student research assistants were opposed at first, on the grounds that the Harvard students who were to be research subjects might not have positive feelings toward Mother Teresa. In fact, some Harvard students had walked out on a commencement address she had given in the 1980s because they disagreed with her strong anti-abortion stance. McClelland was unconcerned about this problem, though. He believed that regardless of whether the students' conscious minds liked Mother Teresa or not, their unconscious minds could not help but respond to the power of her love.

Professor McClelland decided to use a very simple measure of immunity—the secretion rate of an antibody called sIgA in saliva. Like the palace guard, sIgA protects the gates of our body from invasion by bacteria, viruses, and parasites. Deficiencies of sIgA due to intense stress, such as that of a foot soldier in a foxhole or trench, allow a bacterial proliferation in the gums known as *necrotizing gingivitis*—or more aptly—*trench mouth*. Low levels of sIgA would also correlate with more tooth decay and upper respiratory tract infections, such as colds and flu.

Students were asked to spit into test tubes before and after watching Mother Teresa. They also wrote stories in response to a standard set of pictures so that Professor McClelland could get a sample of their thoughts and images with which to score their motives. Sure enough, the film increased both thoughts of unconditional love and the secretion rate of sIgA.

Love, as we discussed in the previous chapter, is a matter of connectedness. In a study that Miron and I did in collaboration with Professor McClelland and one of his former students, Dr. John Jemmott—whose thesis project this was—we found that students whose primary motive was friendship had higher levels of sIgA than those whose primary motive was power. Furthermore, the power-motivated students had dramatic declines in sIgA during exam periods, while those whose primary motive was friendship had much higher levels of sIgA during exams. Friendship, as the studies on the health benefits of social support imply, is good for your health!

Perhaps you've personally experienced feeling better after talking to someone who can understand, through their own experience, what you are going through. Every once in a while I get overtired from traveling and feel like a marathoner who has hit the wall. Although most of my friends can appreciate my feelings of fatigue and empathize with the fact that I'm sick of talking and ready to have a long, solitary rest, I always feel better if I can talk to my friend Loretta, who also travels around the country presenting lectures and workshops. We can exchange funny stories about life on the road from the shared perspective of two women, make plans for how to manage our schedules better, commiserate about our wrinkles, encourage one another's successes, and soothe each other's wounds. By the time I hang up from our conversation, I no longer feel alone. If she can do this, so can I! Even my lymphocytes feel relieved.

CHAPTER SIX

THE MYSTERY CALLED MIND

John was standing by the water cooler at work, laughing at a joke that one of his co-workers had made, when he suddenly doubled over with pain, clutching at his chest. All the breath went out of him, and it seemed as though an enormous weight were crushing his heart. John felt panicked but could not scream or breathe. A minute or so of complete terror seemed to stretch on interminably, but then gave way to the inexplicable presence of overwhelming love and deep peace. John could have rested in that state forever, but a curious thing was happening. He was rising up out of his body, looking down at the peculiar, crumpled form barely recognizable as himself, attended to by one of his co-workers who was administering CPR.

He thought, "Oh, God, I've had a heart attack and I'm dead. But then he thought about all the stories he'd heard about people being resuscitated and reasoned that perhaps he was just having a near-death experience! Perhaps the paramedics would arrive fast enough to save him. As soon as he had that thought, John found himself instantaneously present in the dispatch area where two paramedics were already responding to the call from his office. In a hurry to leave, one of them knocked over a cup of coffee. The paramedics did arrive in time to restart John's heart, and he later validated that, just as he had witnessed while in his out-of-body state, one of them had overturned a styrofoam coffee cup en route to the ambulance.

Over the years, we've heard hundreds of near-death experiences and many of them, like John's, involve specific knowledge of events that were happening some distance away. These stories are intriguing, not only because they clearly demonstrate to us that we are more than our bodies, but also because they lead to speculation on the nature of mind. As medical scientists, we can attest to how little our scientific field understands the powers of the mind.

For the past three chapters, we have been discussing the body/mind without really defining *mind*. Is mind just a random side effect of physiological function—that is, a chance result of electrical fields set up when neurons fire? Are fear and love, delight, and inspiration no more than the mathematical sum of the ion flux that ensues when a neurotransmitter gets squirted out into a synapse? How about the near-death stories? Is the experience of peace, love, and uncommon wisdom—often coupled with the presence of a Supreme Being of Light—merely the meaningless last gasp of oxygen-deprived brain cells? Many scientists such as Carl Sagan and Sir Francis Crick—the latter being the co-discoverer of DNA—believe that it is. Most scientists, in fact, ascribe consciousness to a poorly understood property of neurons.

Personally, we love neurons. Their capacities are incredible. For example, neurons in the right temporal lobe of the brain, when stimulated, will give rise to visions of light. People with temporal lobe epilepsy or TLE, a disorder in which the neurons discharge electrically in an abnormal way, often describe mystic experiences. Another common symptom of TLE is a pressing urge to write material of a religious nature. Some people with TLE complain of orgasmic discharges of energy throughout their body that may even lead to their contortion into yogic postures that they are normally unable to achieve. But does this prove, as some scientists suggest, that all mystics simply had TLE or some other neurological disturbance?

Dr. Melvin Morse, a pediatrician who has written two books— one about near-death experiences in children, and another about light experiences in general—suggests that the right temporal lobe is indeed the "circuit board" for mystical experience. After all, we live in bodies. It is perfectly logical, and consistent with scientific data, to reasonably assume that all of our earthly experiences require some physical circuitry. If the circuitry of the right temporal lobe is stimulated—whether by epilepsy, prolonged meditation, prayer, fasting, drumming, singing, intense joy, intense fear, drugs, or oxygen deprivation—it may be able to process information through newly accessed pathways. There's nothing mysterious about that. After all, every time you turn on your TV or change the channel, you tune into energy waves that were always present in potential form, but simply undecoded until the physical receiver was aligned correctly with the signal.

Miron often points out that if you were mechanically inclined, a TV neurosurgeon, so to speak, you could go into the back of your set and, by severing some wires, you could wipe out your patient's speech. By cutting other wires, you could eliminate the picture or possibly change the nature of the image you see. But does this prove that the signal that comes through your TV—its mind—originates in its circuitry? You can dissect your television thoroughly, and you will never find the little man inside who is reading the news. In terms of the brain, the natural corollary of the opinion that mind resides in the wiring is that when the brain dies, the mind dies, too. What do *you* think? When your TV dies, will the evening news go with it? When your body dies, will the consciousness you know as yourself disappear?

The former Catholic theologian, Caroline Myss, who has the remarkable gift of medical clairvoyance, can diagnose a person's illness without even seeing the individual. Harvard-trained neuroscientist and physician, Norman Shealy, who has studied the mysterious nature of mind for years, validated that Caroline's remote diagnoses were accurate nearly 95 percent of the time. Her accuracy was more impressive than a CAT scan, microscopic laboratory findings, and a physician's finely honed observational skills combined! As scientists, we would hypothesize that the energy waves that each of us continually emanate are encoded with information that

Caroline's brain—or perhaps other cells in her body—can some-how decode.

Neuroreceptor cells in the brain and throughout the body, like televisions, can pick up information through the airwaves. When we see color, for example, we are receiving and decoding energy waves corresponding to a graded spectrum of light. When we hear sound, little hair cells in our inner ears are responding to the magnitude of sound waves. All information is encoded in energy waves. At times, we may receive this information through pathways other than our typical five senses. Such reception is generally called *intuition*.

Intuitive faculties vary from person to person and within the same person at different times. Unlike the well-researched physical senses of seeing, hearing, smelling, touching, and tasting, the intuitive sense of knowing involves physical receptors that our science has yet to discover. But just because the mechanism through which extrasensorial informational energy waves are received is unknown, we cannot infer that no mechanism exists. That would constitute the same kind of "scientific" acumen shown by an 18-month-old child who believes himself to be invisible when a piece of card-board held in front of his eyes shields others from view.

Most of us have had some experience with extrasensory perception. Have you ever thought of a person only to have them telephone a few seconds later? Perhaps you have experienced such a strong sensation that someone in another car was watching you that you felt compelled to turn around and look back. A college friend, "Susan," awoke one night with such a start that she was thrown from her bed. She had dreamed that her fiancé's car had skidded off a steep mountain road. A few hours later, the man's mother called with the terrible news that "Vincent" had indeed died when his car careened over the edge of a steep precipice in the mountains. Susan had been thrown forcefully from her bed at about the same that Vincent had fallen to his death. Was this a coincidence, as some people might argue, or did Vincent and Susan's minds actually touch?

Strong bonds between people, such as the one between Susan and Vincent, or the connection of a mother to her child, seem to predispose one to the extrasensory perception of information. Although I have strong intuition, I certainly don't think of myself as "an intuitive" or psychic. But when our youngest son Andrei was a baby, I left him with Miron one Sunday morning while I went to church. Our kitchen doubled as a family room, and we had placed the baby's playpen several feet from the stove. Although there was ample space between the stove and the playpen, just to be extra safe we never used the playpen if anything was cooking. I had finished pressure-cooking a pot of beans much earlier that morning, so I didn't give a second thought to putting Andrei in the playpen as I walked out the door.

While driving to church about 20 minutes later, I felt a physical "tug" just over my heart where the thymus gland is located. Simultaneously, I saw a vivid vision of the pressure cooker exploding and an arc of hot liquid jetting several feet into the air and hitting Andrei on the right side of his back, just above the diaper line. Confused and upset, I pulled over to think. Was this another example of "awfulizing," or had I really seen something? Should I put a lid on my foolish negative thinking, or should I drive home? Because there is so little support in our culture for intuitive knowing, I concluded that I had been duped by my own negativity. But when I returned home from church a few hours later, an ashen-faced Miron met me at the door. His first words were, "There's been an accident, but don't worry, it's not serious."

I caught my breath and whispered, "Don't tell me. The baby's been burned on his back, hasn't he?" Miron nodded as I ran to Andrei in tears. The freak accident had occurred exactly as I had seen it in the vision. Furthermore, as near as we can tell, I actually saw the vision a few minutes *before* the accident occurred. Andrei was fortunate. Although a few days later the burn had to be debrided, a procedure in which the dead skin is peeled away, the wound healed without incident. In the 21 years that have passed since that Sunday morning, I've never had another precognitive knowing about Andrei or our other two children.

Naturally, I like to believe that if anything serious happened to any family member or close friend, I would get the message, but I can't be sure of that. The sporadic nature of intuitive phenomena points out the precise difficulty in studying them. Although some individuals such as Caroline Myss seem to have a constant receptivity to certain types of information, many of us have only the occasional ability to tune our physiological receptors to extrasensory frequencies.

In the mid-1980s, for example, for no particular reason and with no conscious volition, I developed a fascinating capacity that lasted for only a few weeks. I could guess, to the penny, the amount of change that Miron had in his pocket, or the bill for the groceries. I shocked a few check-out clerks by making out my checks, correct to the penny, before they had even finished totaling up the items in my basket!

For a fascinating review of research in this field, you might enjoy reading *Margins of Reality: The Role of Consciousness in the Physical World,* by Robert Jahn and Brenda Dunne. The book was published in 1987 when Jahn was Professor of Aerospace Sciences and Dean Emeritus of the School of Engineering and Applied Science at Princeton University, and Brenda Dunne was manager of the Princeton Engineering Anomalies Research laboratory, a facility that seeks to extend the margins of science and its understanding of consciousness—the mind.

We hope that this chapter has stimulated you to think a little bit about the nature of the mind. It's heady stuff, if you'll forgive both the pun and the typical tendency to locate the mind in the brain. Each one of us has some conceptualization of mind which, as we will explore in future chapters, has a great deal to do with how we think about life. Those of us who believe that mind is a form of conscious awareness limited in space and time to the vicinity of our brain, subscribe to a *paradigm*, or belief system, resting on separation, isolation, and the ultimate finality of death. Those of us who believe that mind is a form of conscious awareness unlimited by space and time, and shared among all of life—both animate and inanimate—subscribe to a paradigm of interconnectedness that is intimately related to the power of the mind to heal and to the immortality of the soul.

There is no time when our understanding of the mystery of mind has been more important, for at no other point in history did we have sufficient knowledge to destroy ourselves and our planet. On a hopeful note, Caroline Myss believes that our species is undergoing an actual physical transformation from *Homo sapiens* to *Homo noeticus*. The former term means "man of knowledge"—a very valuable, but somewhat limited, form of knowing based only on reason. The latter term means "man of intuition"—capable of the direct perception of information that is unlimited by bias, belief, space, or time.

This evolution in consciousness may indeed involve an actual physical change in the right temporal lobe of our brains. It is interesting to note that one in twenty Americans, or more than eight million people, have had near-death experiences. And about 20 percent of those have subsequently reported fascinating changes in their ability to perceive information and interact with the physical world.

One such change is electrical sensitivity. Such "electrical sensitives" can no longer wear watches, because something about their energy field actually stops their operation. Many such people also report the nonintentional shutting down of computers, street lights, and electrical appliances as they walk by! Other phenomena may include the development of intuition and other special abilities such as medical clairvoyance, contact with angelic realms, and the power to heal by the laying-on of hands. Is it possible that the right temporal lobe activity of these "sensitives" was changed by the near-death experience?

Fortunately, we don't have to undergo a near-death experience to open up the limitless possibilities of our minds. As we shall examine, the power of prayer, meditation, belief, and basic good-heartedness can all put us in touch with a reality much richer than our current science can describe. Then, perhaps, we can realize intuitively what the great quantum physicist Erwin Schrodinger meant when he commented that if we could measure the sum total of all the minds that were present in the Universe, there would be just *one*.

CHAPTER SEVEN

THE MEETING OF THE MINDS

I'm one of those people who generally avoids enclosed shopping malls because they induce a kind of mild anxiety. The lack of fresh air, the strong fluorescent lighting, and the overwhelming assault of color and sound can make anyone a little anxious. But what if, in addition to these obvious properties, some of us feel a bit peculiar in malls and other crowded places because, at a subliminal level, we pick up the constant chatter of other people's thoughts, desires, and judgments?

One afternoon in the mid-1970s, while still an assistant professor at Tufts Medical School, I went shopping during my lunch hour. The Tufts medical area is a short walk from the heart of downtown Boston and the once-renowned bargain-hunter's paradise, Filene's Basement. Intent on checking out what was billed as a blockbuster sweater sale, I made my way through the crowds, down the long flight of stairs under Filene's, and arrived at the basement, instantly anxious and overwhelmed. But after several measured, deep breaths, I was able to relax a little and press on. Ever the intrepid shopper, I was determined to get to that sale!

The deep breathing helped me distance myself from the anxiety, and I began to think about why I felt so upset. As if in answer to that mental question, songs started to go through my mind. The Everly brothers were just beginning *Dream, Dream, Dream*—but before they could finish, a Christian spiritual whose words were foreign to me cut across the mental airwaves. A Beatles song came in next, followed by what felt like a brief rush of greed. The entire experience lasted for perhaps a minute, during which time I felt a combination of fear, curiosity, and vulnerability. Remembering an old meditation exercise consisting of enclosing oneself in an egg of light, I mentally created a cocoon of safety and privacy. The music stopped, and I felt safer and more spacious. The blue sweater I bought that day is long gone, but the memory of being swept away in a tide of other's people's thoughts still remains.

Our body/mind, which naturally includes our thoughts, is composed of electrical wave-energy that is still unnamed by Western science. There are, however, names for this life-force energy in many different cultures. It is called *Qi* (pronounced *chi*) in China, *Ki* in Japan, and *shakti* or *kundalini* in India. Practitioners of martial arts such as aikido consciously work with their own life-force energy as well as that of their opponent. The martial arts are, in their purest form, mental arts. Yoga, too, is a form of mental control of the body's vital energy.

That day in Filene's Basement, I used the egg-of-light meditation, a form of mental martial arts (which you will learn at the end of this chapter), to protect myself from the adverse effects of other people's thought energy. The *shamans*, or indigenous healers, from many cultures share the belief that an energy field emanates from all living things. And for many of them, the energy body is not a belief; it is an observable reality. They can experience it just as clearly as I could hear other people's intrusive musical interludes and sense their desires. The balance of this vital energy is considered a key aspect for both physical and emotional well-being.

Physician and researcher Dr. David Eisenberg has been studying Chinese medicine since 1977. His interest was piqued originally by the reports of James Reston, a reporter for the *New York Times*, who underwent an emergency appendectomy under acupuncture-induced anesthesia while accompanying Nixon and his party to Beijing in 1971. Eisenberg studied the Chinese language while an undergraduate, and honed it during long periods of study and shorter visits to China, both during and after completing his medical training at Harvard. In 1985 Eisenberg led a group of colleagues from Harvard Medical School on a fact-finding tour to Shanghai and Beijing. I was fortunate to be a part of that group and to have had the opportunity to meet both with Chinese scientists and Qi masters.

The Chinese believe that the Qi can be moved internally via subtle energy channels called *meridians* through the practice of breathing exercises, mental concentration, and the meditative movements known as *t'ai qi chu'an* (tai chi). By 6:00 A.M. every morning, we were amazed to see literally thousands of Chinese citizens of every age practicing this ancient art of well-being in unison in the public parks. Qi can also be directed externally—moved from one person to another. The ability to control the flow of Qi is called *Qi Gong*, literally, "the manipulation of vital energy."

Qi Gong masters have traditionally demonstrated their control of the vital forces in many of the same ways as Indian yogic adepts. In some demonstrations, yogis have reclined on a bed of sharp nails that would ordinarily pierce the skin. In different variations of this performance, they are subsequently jumped on, run over by a truck, or weighted down by concrete blocks. Upon arising from the bed of nails, their skin is completely unmarked! Qi Gong masters give similar demonstrations, some of which we were privileged to see while in China.

When I was a college student, I saw a demonstration that stymied me until I saw it repeated 20 years later in a small village a few hours' drive outside of Shanghai. Just before the end of the school year one May, a traveling circus had come to one of the Main Line Philadelphia towns near Bryn Mawr, where I was a student. One of the side shows featured a handsome, muscular young black man who could "control the life energy." I was fascinated by the performer's precise, fluid movements—a kind of feline grace, and by his calm presence.

I'd been expecting circus hype, but the young yogi went quietly about his business. Dumping approximately 50 glass Coca-Cola bottles out of a sack, he set about smashing them with a sledgehammer. He then invited us to examine the broken glass. I picked up a shard and promptly punctured my thumb. It was definitely the real thing. He then invited us to examine the soles of his bare feet. They were smooth and soft, certainly no more callused than my own. After closing his eyes and taking a few deep breaths, the young man proceeded to jump up and down vigorously on the glass for at least two minutes. At the end of the demonstration, when we examined his feet, they were as smooth and unmarred as they had been before.

I was amazed by this demonstration and was unable to figure out any rational explanation for it. But then, magicians such as Doug Henning can seemingly make elephants disappear. It's important not to underestimate the power of suggestion and belief in creating powerful illusions. But when we saw precisely the same glass-jumping demonstration in rural China, conducted as part of a scientific demonstration rather than as a circus amusement, I was amazed anew by the remarkable power of the mind. Certainly these sincere Chinese government scientists had no intention of duping their American colleagues with magic tricks!

In China the practice of external Qi Gong—in which the master's powers are directed toward others—has a 3,000-year-old history. This phenomenon is a venerable one even though scientific investigations just began in 1978, only a few years after the introduction of acupuncture in the West. Western scientists first relegated acupuncture to the "trash heap" of the placebo effect, its efficacy written off as suggestion. But when researchers demonstrated that acupuncture anesthesia worked on donkeys, the suggestion hypothesis began to lose some of its luster! A large volume of studies subsequently documented the efficacy of acupuncture, not only for certain types of anesthesia and pain control, but also for the treatment of conditions as diverse as cystic breasts and hypertension. Similar research is now being done with external Qi Gong.

While in China, some members of our party witnessed a Qi master transferring energy to a fluorescent bulb that he was holding. Although the bulb was not plugged in, he succeeded in lighting it, following a moment or two of breathing exercises! In the same way, Qi can be directed at a patient undergoing surgery to stimulate key acupuncture points without the use of needles. The Chinese believe that this Qi energy is responsible not only for physical health, but for telepathy, clairvoyance, and psychokinesis—the ability to cause the movement of objects without touching them.

Such energetic phenomena, which have long been accepted in other cultures, pose a challenge to Western scientific thinking, which is lacking in the notion of a vital force. If external Qi Gong is possible, it leads to an interesting question: While there is no scientific doubt that our minds affect our own bodies, might it also be true that our minds can affect other people's bodies as well?

Some well-known experiments in quantum physics suggest that we may, indeed, be able to influence one another at a distance. They suggest, in fact, that a universal energy connects all things— no matter how separate they might appear—and that this energy transcends the limitations of time and space.

In 1964, a quantum physicist by the name of John Stewart Bell reported an experiment with mind-boggling implications. His data implied that once two particles have been in contact with one another, they remain connected—and are capable of influencing one another—even if they migrate to opposite ends of the Universe! Bell's Theorem states that one atom of a molecule somehow "knows" what another atom it was once paired with is doing. This "knowing" does not rely on forms of energy such as light, sound, or gravity that decrease over distance. In other words, the form of energy that underlies these phenomena is not localized in space or time, but is nonlocal. It acts across great distances.

Physician and author Dr. Larry Dossey has introduced the terms *local* and *nonlocal* mind to discuss the relation of quantum physics to the power of the mind to heal. His excellent books, *Space, Time and Medicine*; *Recovering the Soul;* and *Healing Words* present a compelling and readable description of the intersection between the strange, anomalous world of quantum physics, nonlocal phenomena, and healing—what he calls "a world behind the scenes."

Consider the implications of Bell's Theorem. It is well known that our apparently solid world of people, trees, smokestacks, and dogs is made up of a veritable beehive of busy atoms all in perpetual motion. We can liken the solid human body to the night sky, in which every visible star is like an atom. Most of the sky—like most of our bodies and all things—is made up of empty space. Atoms zip in and out of that space constantly. An atom that was in your brain tissue last week may well be part of the gut of a chicken next week. Molecules in the wing of a fly may recycle into your bone tissue. Atoms that were once part of Mahatma Ghandi, Mother Teresa, Jesus Christ, Adolph Hitler, and Attila the Hun are still cycling in and out of every one of us. If Bell's Theorem is correct, and at some level all those atoms stay perpetually connected, then in some way, we are all always connected. We share an enormous data bank of experience.

Of course, there is still controversy among physicists as to the validity of Bell's Theorem. Some believe that it will stand as research progresses, while others believe that some other explanation for his results will eventually be found. In the meantime, we can look to a scientific principle known as *parsimony* to predict whether Bell will be proven right or wrong. Parsimony means simplicity. Generally speaking, the most basic explanation that can account for diverse results turns out to be the correct one. Bell's Theorem is simple, and it can account for phenomena that many people have experienced, although our science considers them anomalous or impossible.

Gallup polls and the National Social Survey conducted by the University of Chicago's National Opinion Research Council indicate that the majority of Americans routinely experience phenomena consistent with a nonlocal model of mind. Surveys conducted in 1973 and then repeated in the mid-1980s indicate that the incidence and variety of experiences ranging from contact with dead relatives to déjà vu have risen sharply in recent years. Nearly one-third of the American public reported having visions in the mid-1980s, as opposed to only 8 percent in 1973! Fully half of all adults believe that they have had contact with the dead, up from 25 percent in 1973. And a whopping two-thirds of people reported extrasensory perception, up from 58 percent in the earlier survey.

Until fairly recently, people have argued that experiences of nonlocal mind might indicate psychosis or other mental illness, which is one reason why (as these topics have become more socially acceptable) the apparent incidence may have risen. Perhaps we are simply more comfortable talking about experiences that might previously have been judged as unbalanced or "far out." Or perhaps, as Caroline Myss suggests, we are actually undergoing an evolution as a species in the ability to perceive more of the reality in which we live.

Priest, sociologist, author, and researcher Father Andrew Greeley investigated people who had mystical visions to find out what they had in common. His findings do away with the hypothesis that people who have such experiences are either religious fanatics or candidates for locked wards. His research indicated that people who have nonlocal encounters tend to be quite ordinary, slightly above average in education and intelligence, and a bit below the median in religious involvement. When tested psychologically, they scored at the top of the scale for healthy personalities.

Now, while experiences of nonlocal mind may be common, the challenge is to demonstrate scientifically that we can affect one another with our thoughts. A fascinating experiment conducted at the Mind Science Foundation in San Antonio, Texas, shows just that. Researchers William Braud and Marilyn Schlitz did 13 separate experiments in which a total of 271 volunteers from the community were hooked up to sensitive biofeedback equipment that monitored their level of tension or relaxation. The individual ability of a total of 62 other volunteers to influence their tension or relaxation levels at a distance was assessed. The influencers were instructed to either try to calm or excite the research subjects, who were in a distant room, by creating mental images of tension or relaxation for themselves and then strongly intending to send those images to the subject, while also imagining the output of the biofeedback equipment moving in the desired direction.

The subjects had no idea whether they were being sent calming or exciting thoughts, and yet they responded to these mental intentions consistently and reliably from trial to trial at a level that reached statitistical significance. Many subjects reported picking up specific images that the influencer had, in fact, sent.

These experiments indicate that the ability to influence others with our mental images at a distance is common, rather than confined to a few people with special ability. As Larry Dossey has noted, this is both good news and bad news. On the positive side, he comments in *Healing Words* that "Subjects with a greater need to be influenced—that is, those for whom the influence would be beneficial—seem more susceptible," and also that "the transpersonal imagery effect is not invariable. Subjects appear capable of shielding or preventing the effect if it is unwanted."

Do you have friends or family in whose presence you feel particularly peaceful, while others make you nervous or seem to suck the energy right out of you? Many cultures recommend variants of the following egg-of-light exercise to shield your energy body from being polluted by other people's thoughts, and to protect other people from being harmed by your thoughts.

Try reading this exercise through once or twice and noting the main points. Then give it a try. We recommend using it every morning when you get up. You may wish to tape it for yourself, repeating the directions slowly until the exercise becomes second nature. Pause briefly at the dots until you have *experienced or imagined* what the instructions say.

EGG-OF-LIGHT EXERCISE

Begin by taking a good stretch, and then allow your eyes to close.... Focus lightly on your breathing, noticing the way that your body rises slightly as you breathe in and relaxes down as you breathe out....As you settle gently into observing the tide of your incoming and outgoing breath, your concentration can become more and more focused....

Now, in the space above you and slightly in front of you, imagine a great star of loving light....Allow the light to cascade over you like a waterfall and to run through you....Imagine the light entering the top of your head and running down through and between every cell, the way that a river washes through the sand on its bottom.... Allow the river of light to carry away any fatigue, illness, or negativity and wash it out through the bottoms of your feet into the earth for transformation....

As the river of light washes through you, imagine that it is scrubbing away any darkness around your heart, allowing the light within you to shine more and more brightly....joining with the river of light....filling you and extending around you for two or three feet in every direction like an enormous, luminous egg....

Make a firm mental declaration that any thoughts of love and encouragement will penetrate the egg and reach your heart, while any negative thoughts will bounce off the egg and return to the sender as a blessing. Declare also that your own loving thoughts will penetrate the egg and reach their destination, while your negative thoughts will bounce off the interior of the egg and return you to the awareness of lovingkindness and encouragement.

Anytime during the day that you feel anxious, assaulted by someone's energy, or fatigued, try the egg-of-light exercise. After you are used to doing it, you can place yourself in the egg almost instantaneously.

CHAPTER EIGHT

HEALING AND NONLOCAL MIND

Just before Christmas of 1992, I had the unique opportunity of appearing on *Geraldo* (the popular daytime talk show) as "an expert on miracles." While I don't claim that title myself, the producers assigned it to me so that I could comment on the fascinating experiences of a diverse group of panelists. They ranged from a woman who had been healed at Lourdes; to a bright, energetic young boy who had been dying from liver failure and transplant-related pneumonia when his mother begged the local newspaper to publish a plea for readers to pray for him. The paper estimated that more than a million people prayed for the child. Contrary to medical expectations, the boy made a rapid recovery within 48 hours. According to his mother, the hospital referred to her son as "their little Easter miracle."

Many physicians are fascinated by the occurrence of such healings but blanch at the word *miracle* because it seems unscientific. In his superb book, *Recovering the Soul: A Scientific and Spiritual Search*, Dr. Larry Dossey provides an astute scientific framework that can house both medicine and miracles. Dr. Dossey outlines three eras, or epochs, in our understanding of medicine.

Era 1 is the scientific medicine we know today, which is still in its infancy. This era of mechanical medicine, which views the body as a machine, began to burgeon in the late 19th century. Based on a growing understanding of the cause of disease, specific cures could be found. In 1907, for example, Dr. Paul Ehrlich discovered that the great scourge of syphilis could be cured with arsenic. This was one of the first "magic bullets," a specific treatment that could wipe out a dread disease. In the years that followed, other magic bullets were discovered. Vitamin C was found to cure scurvy, and insulin-replacement therapy allowed diabetics to live normal lives. By World War II, the sulfa drugs were commonly used to treat wound infections that might have been lethal in earlier times. Immunosuppressive drugs now allow for organ transplants that make the body-as-machine analogy a reality. Era I is a powerful, life-enhancing, life-saving form of medicine.

Era ll medicine is the mind/body approach. As I learned from my stress-related illnesses in graduate school, sometimes we cannot be cured by magic bullets. Studies indicate that about 80 percent of all visits to primary care physicians are for stress-related diseases or problems such as colds or flu that will go away on their own. Only a minority of ills require the magic bullets of Era 1 medicine. Until modern medicine came along, of course, mind/body medicine was well understood. The more subtle effects of belief, however, were overshadowed by the great breakthroughs in modern treatment. Only as we slowly began to realize some of the limitations of Era 1 has there been a resurgence of interest in the power of the mind to heal.

Era lll medicine represents a quantum leap in the useful but incomplete paradigm upon which the first two eras are based. Era 1 medicine is based on the metaphor of body-as-machine, yet Era ll is no less mechanistic. Most of the research in mind/body medicine, for example, really investigates the brain/body connection. Mind is still thought of as a local, mortal function of brain activity. Era lll medicine is, in Dossey's words, "a radical departure from this model," an opening into a world that is unlimited by space and time. Healing through prayer is an example of nonlocal mind acting on the body at a distance.

Caroline Myss' stunning record of remote diagnosis is another Era lll phenomenon, as is the occurrence of telesomatic illness. Do you remember my college friend Susan whom we discussed previously? When her sleeping body was thrown from bed half a world away from where her fiancé Vincent's car was hurtling over a cliff, a nonlocal telesomatic event was occurring.

The word *telesomatic* is derived from the Greek *tele*, meaning *far off,* and *somatikos*, meaning *body*. Telesomatic events, according to Dr. Dossey, are relatively common. For example, a son in New York has an episode of excruciating chest pain only to find that his father has just died of a heart attack in Boston. Telesomatic events seem to rely, in part, on an empathic bond between the people involved. While reading some of the research studies, I was struck by the way that we bear one another's pain, how we suffer together.

I have personally experienced two or three very brief episodes of depression during which I felt disorganized, unmotivated, and hopeless. These, I believe, were telesomatic events in which I picked up depression from other family members. In effect, I acted out their symptoms. Several of my patients have similarly complained of functioning as psychic sponges at times. The natural corollary of telesomatic illness, however, is telesomatic healing. There may be times when we feel uncharacteristically insightful, patient, compassionate, forgiving, or cheerful only to realize that a loved one has been working hard on their own healing, and we are reaping some of the benefits! The physics underlying nonlocality predicts what spiritual teachers from many traditions have said: *Whenever any person heals, the whole community is uplifted.*

The potential healing effects of prayer, the ability to diagnose at a distance, and telesomatic illness and healing definitely challenge the Era 1 world view of body-as-machine and mind as an emergent function of that machine. Yet, physicians and scientists are no less conversant with these possibilities than the rest of us; they are simply less comfortable discussing what can appear to be unscientific. In the late 1980s, I decided to break that medical silence at a meeting of obstetrician/gynecologists who had invited me to update them on psychoneuroimmunology and the body/mind connection.

I was feeling frisky, so I asked the conference attendees whether they wanted my tame slides or my wild mind! They were tired. They'd seen a lot of slides and were ready for a break, so they opted for wild mind. We had a fascinating afternoon discussing near-death experiences, healing at a distance, and the few scientific studies that have been conducted on prayer. I was half expecting to dodge a volley of rotten tomatoes, if not a visit from the heresy police, but I was pleasantly surprised.

After the lecture, a group of physicians stood in line for over an hour to share cases in which prayer had resulted in miraculous healings. A reception followed, and I've never heard such excited discussion as these physicians recounted their personal experiences of nonlocal mind. One doctor told me that he'd known that consciousness was more than brain function since college. One night at a frat party he had drunk enough to induce alcohol poisoning. When he went back to his room and got into bed, he found himself floating above his body, accurately seeing details of the room clearly above the vantage point of his physical eyes.

In his fine book, *Healing Words: The Power of Prayer and the Practice of Medicine*, Dr. Dossey ably reconciles science and prayer in part through a careful investigation of all the studies that have been conducted on the subject of prayer. There are a couple of very interesting ones. Perhaps the most famous of them was published in the *Southern Medical Journal* in July of 1988 by a cardiologist, Dr. Randolph Byrd, who was working at the San Francisco General Hospital. He conducted a randomized, controlled, double-blind study—the gold standard of good science.

Four hundred patients who were admitted to the coronary intensive-care unit with a heart attack or suspected heart attack were assigned to one of two groups: standard intensive care only, or intensive care plus prayer at a distance. Groups of people who met for the purpose of prayer were given the names of the patients and told a little bit about their condition. Each patient had first signed an informed consent form that specified that they had an equal chance of being prayed for. They could, of course, pray for themselves, or their friends and relatives could pray for them. But with such a large number of people in the study, the laws of chance are such that all other prayer being equal, the specific variable in the study would be the extra prayer from the prayer groups.

Since the study was double-blind, neither the patients nor the staff knew who was being prayed for. This is critical, since if you knew you were being prayed for and if you believed in prayer, you would definitely improve due to the placebo effect—a powerful phenomenon in which your own mind is affecting your body. If the hospital staff knew who was being prayed for, they might have given preferential treatment to one or the other group. So, the double-blind model is an important aspect of this research.

Dr. Byrd found that the prayed-for group fared significantly better than the nonprayed-for group on several counts: They were less likely to develop congestive heart failure and pulmonary edema (where the lungs fill with fluid); they were five times less likely to require antibiotics; fewer needed to be put on ventilators and receive artificial respiration; even fewer developed pneumonia or had cardiac arrests; and fewer died, although this last finding was not statistically significant.

In addition to a handful of studies involving human beings, there is a somewhat larger body of literature that reveals how simpler life forms have been subjected to prayer. Some of the most interesting findings come from the Spindrift Foundation in Lansdale, Pennsylvania, whose purpose is the scientific study of prayer. Some of their early studies involved seeds soaked in salt water to inhibit germination. When such seeds were prayed for, significantly more of the prayed-for seeds germinated compared to unprayed-for controls. (In fact, if you want to replicate this study, you can write to Spindrift for a home prayer study kit at the address in the resource section at the back of this book!)

The Spindrift researchers make a point of distinguishing between directed and nondirected prayer. Directed prayer specifies a particular outcome, such as increased germination. The spiritual healer Agnes Sanford calls this "scientific" prayer and specifies how to go about it in her classic book, *The Healing Light*. It is a three-step process that involves (1) feeling a connection to the mind of God that is in all things, (2) seeing the results of the prayer as already accomplished, and (3) giving thanks. She hastens to say, however, that if our prayers are not in accordance with Divine will, nothing will come of them. Nondirected prayer is what the Spindrift researchers call a "pure and holy qualitative consciousness of whoever or whatever is being prayed for." Rather than having a specific goal, it is a prayer for the highest good or for the best potential to manifest. In the Spindrift experiments, both types of prayer were successful in increasing gemination.

The philosopher and psychologist Erich Fromm once said that a good mother looks upon her child with a "passion for the possible." What a great definition of nondirected prayer! In a Harvard study, teachers were given a list of students who were supposed to be ready to make great strides academically according to test results. In fact, the list of their names had been chosen at random. But at the end of the year, those students had blossomed. Their best potential had indeed expressed itself. It may be that the teachers looked for any sign of success and encouraged it outwardly. But perhaps the results were also related to the encouraging mental image they held of these students—a form of nondirected prayer.

Stop and reflect for a moment. Think about your family members, friends and the people you interact with on the job. Are your thoughts about them loving and encouraging, or they are limiting and critical? You don't have to believe in God or invoke a Higher Power to be praying. Every thought and attitude is a kind of prayer.

> *Read the rest of this paragraph, and then try this exercise before going on. Take a nice stretch, and then allow your eyes to close. Begin to focus your mind by paying attention to your breathing. Notice the way that your body rises gently as you breathe in, and how it relaxes down as you breathe out....Now, bring a family member or friend to mind in as much detail as you can. Imagine that you can look deeply into his or her eyes, directly to their*

soul....See the beauty and creative promise in this person. Mentally encourage their potential, affirming "What a talented, loving person you really are." If you feel inspired, do this exercise for a few more people.

When I was a cancer cell biologist at Tufts Medical School, I had a good friend who was a clinical cancer specialist. During those years, I was collecting journal articles and case studies about the small number of people who had spontaneous remissions from cancer. "Dave" used to laugh at me when we discussed these unexpected healings. His point of view was that if cancer could be cut out or burned out before it had spread, you were lucky. Your good luck extended to chemotherapy for Hodgkin's disease and a few other lymphomas. But in all other cases, Dave believed, if the cancer had spread, you were going to die. He was sure that spontaneous remissions were all misdiagnoses. Even though Dave was an extremely caring, gentle man, would you want him to be your oncologist? Think about the "prayers" that his limited thinking represent.

Some patients have told me that they have a certain sense about their doctor, an intuition that goes beyond the physician's bedside manner or the decor in the office. One woman told me that she couldn't help thinking of her oncologist as Dr. Death, an eponym that predated the appearance of Dr. Jack Kevorkian (who is well known for helping patients die through assisted suicide). If your intuition tells you that you are visiting Dr. Death, don't worry about people-pleasing or standing on formalities. Resign from the relationship, and seek out a doctor who feels life-affirming to you. Our friend and colleague Dr. Bernie Siegel says that most people invest more time picking out a new car than they do in finding a doctor upon whom their life may depend. The respect, hope, and encouragement of health professionals are prayers that allow the power of their minds to help us heal.

CHAPTER NINE

WHAT'S A BODY TO DO?
Wise Choices for Healing

Once upon a time there was a farmer who believed firmly in the power of prayer. One morning a flood swept through the rural community where he lived, an event that occasioned impassioned prayers for help. When the water had risen to his bottom windows, a neighbor arrived in a rowboat to bring him to safety. The farmer declined, saying "God will save me." When the water had risen to the second story of the farmer's house, another neighbor came by in a powerful motorboat. Once again the farmer declined rescue: "Thanks anyway. God will save me."

By early evening, the farmer was standing resolutely on his chimney when a helicopter flew overhead and let down a rope. The farmer waved it away, smiling. "God will save me." A few minutes later, he found himself face to face with St. Peter at the Pearly Gates. Confused and disillusioned, he shook his head. "Why didn't you save me? Didn't God hear my prayers?"

St. Peter laughed till he cried. "You are so stubborn! We sent a rowboat, a motorboat, and a helicopter. What more could we do?"

Sometimes, as was the case with the farmer, our opinions blind us to the obvious. I once gave a lecture at the renowned Chautaqua summer community in New York State. In the 1800s a network of 2,500 Chautaquas—summer communities for the study of art, music and religion—spanned the country. While all but three of these have disappeared, the New York Chautaqua is a venerable institution and a thriving summer community of nearly 10,000 people. It was thrilling to deliver a Sunday lecture on healing to nearly 4,000 people there. I was particularly excited to feel the buzz of electricity that passed through the audience as we began to talk about the healing power of prayer.

When it was time for the question-and-answer period, someone asked my opinion about the famous Twitchell case. The Twitchells were Christian Scientists whose young son had developed severe belly pain. In accordance with their beliefs, they called a Christian Science practitioner to pray for the boy, who subsequently died from a bowel obstruction that could have been effectively treated by Era 1 medicine. I can't imagine the pain that these parents endured—parents who clearly loved their child but who were also devout believers in the exclusive use of the power of prayer for healing. Their family's tragedy led to nationwide concern about how we ought to choose our medical treatments and what our responsibility might be to others who, by virtue of age or mental status, cannot make such decisions for themselves.

I told the story of the farmer and the flood to summarize, in a sense, my feelings on the Twitchell case. If God, or some Universal Force, created everything, why isn't medicine also an answer to our prayers? When we're marooned on our chimney with cancer, who's to say that the surgeon is not divinely guided? For me, using both prayer and medicine poses no moral dilemma. My paternal grandmother was both a Jew and a Christian Scientist who modeled a flexible approach to life. When she or someone else in the family was ill, she called the doctor. She also called her friends, and together they prayed.

There are times when one of the three eras of medicine may be preferable because it is most efficacious, but the three can often be used together. In 1987, I fell asleep at the wheel of my car, and a serious head-on collision resulted in my nose being opened and nearly severed. At the scene of the accident, I prayed (Era lll) and also used mental imagery for healing and relaxation (Era ll). I had no illusions, however, about imagining or praying for my nose to be put back into place. As soon as the ambulance pulled into the hospital where I was on staff, I had the Emergency Room nurse page Joel, their most technically competent Era 1 plastic surgeon. As it happened, he was much more than a brilliant surgeon. During the examination, Joel gently inquired as to whether the metaphor "life in the fast lane" applied to me. Sadly, the most applicable metaphor was really "falling asleep at the wheel" of my life. At that time, life was running *me*, and I felt seriously out of control.

Before this wonderful physician injected the Novocaine and began reconstructing my face, he asked whether I wished to pray. When I said yes, he announced that he would pray, too. I felt profoundly touched and cared for. As the surgery progressed, he gave my body/mind powerful suggestions for healing which, he said, was a natural function of the body. Healing, according to Joel, was as simple as breathing. Complete recovery would follow as long as I stayed out of nature's way. Staying out of the way included avoiding activities that might raise blood pressure, thus congesting damaged tissue. It also included minimizing emotional stress. While Joel knew that I taught stress reduction, he wanted to be sure that I was fully capable of staying home from work for a month, resting in bed, letting people help, and saying no to demands on my time.

At each follow-up appointment, Joel would shake his head and smile, assuring me that the healing was going well and remarking that we had a silent partner—God. Healing required the communion and commitment of all three of us—Joel, myself, and that unknown Creative Spirit. It wasn't until 18 months after the accident, when my nose was looking great after a second surgery, that Joel revealed the full extent of the injury. In 12 years of big-city emergency surgery, the damage to my nose was the worst Joel had ever seen. On a scale of one to 10, where 10 was complete destruction, my nose rated an 8. You'd never know it now. That revelation increased my awe of the body's capacity to heal when conditions are optimal.

In distinct contrast to Joel, who was a healer in the truest sense of the word, Dr. X was a surgeon whom I consulted for a period of years about lumps in my breast. He was technically competent and very kind, but didn't subscribe to the partnership notion of healing. Ever the authority, he could barely prevent himself from scoffing when I arrived for a check-up because of a dream I'd had.

In the dream, I was clutching a bottle of nitroglycerin over my right breast. I got to the hospital just in time for a nurse to pour it down the drain before it could explode. Upon awakening, I could still feel a strong sensation of heat in my breast. I tend to be the sort of person who avoids doctors and has a wait-and-see attitude about symptoms, but after two or three more breast dreams, I believed that the unconscious wisdom of the body might be trying to give me an important message.

Dr. X gave me a short lecture on managing anxiety and suggested rather sarcastically, since he knew that I ran support groups for people with cancer and other illnesses, that I might want to find a support group for women with cancer phobia. I felt that his response was really motivated by kindness. He was trying, in his own way, to convince me that I had absolutely nothing to worry about since no lumps were palpable, and my annual mammograms were clear.

On the previous two mammograms, however, a small calcium deposit had shown up. During my next mammogram, several months after Dr. X had dismissed my dream, one of the radiologists at the hospital suggested that if I wanted, I could have the calcification biopsied. Although it was almost certainly nothing to worry about, some other patterns of calcification were associated with malignancy. I laughed. "Who'd want a biopsy for nothing? I'm not the nervous sort."

After a week or two had elapsed, however, the nitroglycerin dream came strongly to mind. I decided to consult with a well-known female breast surgeon, Dr. Susan Love, whose *Breast Book* is a must for all women. Susan turned out to be the kind of physician who is a true partner in healing. Although she, too, thought it unlikely that the calcification was serious, she still thought it best to take it out. Susan drew me a very helpful diagram of how—and over what time period—normal cells transform into cancerous cells. The process actually takes years and is reversible at several points. She also outlined the various treatment options we would have at our disposal in the unlikely case that the calcification was malignant.

As surgeries go, everything went smoothly. I walked into the operating room on my own two feet, and was even allowed to keep my shoes on! Susan, her scrub nurse, and I carried on a nonstop conversation during the procedure, and when the surgery was over, I got up and walked back out of the operating room. Susan and the other professionals had done a great service without making me feel weak, dependent, or sick. I felt like a friend and colleague rather than a patient. When Susan called to tell me that the calcification had indeed been precancerous, but not yet malignant, I breathed a sigh of relief. The "nitroglycerin" had been poured down the drain before it could explode.

In his excellent book, *The Healing Path*, health writer Mark Barasch documents his own journey of healing from a thyroid cancer that he also discovered on account of a series of dreams. Barasch comments that "healing implies a restoration of communication with ourselves." If we're present to ourselves, the body's inner wisdom lets us know what we need. Small children, for example, can be trusted to choose a balanced diet—not day by day—but week by week. Even though they may eat only macaroni one day and fruit the next, they are responding to physiological signals from the body/mind. As we get older, these signals get obscured in different ways. Excessive use of sugar and caffeine dulls our receptivity to the body's messages, as do nicotine, alcohol, and other drugs.

Similarly, denial of emotional pain blocks communication between the body/mind and our conscious knowing. After all, emotions are literally a "felt sense" within the body. Anxiety can feel like butterflies in the stomach, rapid heartbeat, or muscle tension. Peace feels deeply relaxing. Love is a sense of the heart and throat opening. But if we block painful feelings, we also shut off the ability to sense enjoyable ones.

If there is reduced conscious awareness of the body's needs, information is likely to come through the unconscious. Many people have reported that the first inkling of illness came through a dream or a "knowing." A social worker we knew was researching ovarian cancer when she felt a strong intuition that she, too, had the disease. An ultrasound confirmed the presence of a suspicious mass that did, indeed, turn out to be cancer.

There is a fine line, though, between intuition and hypochondria! Distinguishing between important communication from the unconscious mind and plain old awfulizing is something that takes practice. My own rule of thumb about dreams, for instance, is that when one awakens with a very strong physical or emotional sensation, the dream is likely to be important. Its importance is underscored when similar themes recur in subsequent dreams.

Appropriate health care, then, relies on your ability to communicate with your own wisdom, as well as with the team of professionals you hire to help you. The optimal time to look for a good doctor who will work in partnership with you is not when a bona fide emergency arises or when you intuit that you may be ill. Walking into the average doctor's office for an initial check-up because of something you dreamed is likely to set off "here comes a weirdo" alarm bells. *It's best to find a good physician when you are well,* and establish a relationship. A physician needs to know you as a person before he or she can get a good sense of what your symptoms may represent.

In addition to having a competent, respectful Era 1 physician, you may wish to consult homeopaths, naturopaths, massage therapists, acupuncturists, or other "alternative" practitioners. Just as you would ask for the credentials of a prospective allopath (Western-trained physician), you would want to be informed about the training of alternative practitioners. An acupuncturist trained for four years in China has considerably more expertise than one trained for a year in the U.S. And just as you would prefer an allopathic ally who is open to other forms of healing, good alternative healers will also be open to allopathic medicine. Partnership, rather than exclusivity, sets the stage for healing.

During the time that I directed the Mind/Body Clinic, a woman whom I'll call "Alice" came to see me about symptoms including fatigue, anxiety, feelings of worthlessness, and poor sleep. She was clearly clinically depressed. In the previous six months, Alice had seen an acupuncturist who believed that he could cure her symptoms, but there was no relief. An iridologist (an iris specialist) who diagnosed Alice's problems by looking in her eyes had recommended hundreds of dollars' worth of nutritional supplements, but these also failed her. She had tried hatha yoga and colonic cleansings, all to no avail. Now Alice wanted to join the mind/body program because she felt that meditation might help. Instead, I referred her to a psychiatrist for evaluation of her depression.

When I told Alice that imbalances in brain biochemistry sometimes needed to be corrected through antidepressants before a person could even begin to meditate, she got furious with me. Here she had come for Era ll medicine, and I was pushing Era 1 pharmacology! I didn't hear from her for about six months and assumed that she wouldn't be back. But one day, a very perky Alice arrived for another appointment.

After our first meeting, she had continued to try alternatives. Polarity therapy (a kind of energy balancing) and Chinese herbs had made no difference. Finally, when Alice began to feel suicidal, the prospect of visiting a psychiatrist seemed not only reasonable, but critical. He prescribed Imipramine, a standard tricyclic antidepressant, and within three weeks she felt like her old self. Now Alice felt ready to begin the clinical program of meditation and the development of insight that I described in my first book, *Minding the Body, Mending the Mind.*

All of the alternative treatments that Alice tried have been known to be helpful, but usually not for clinical depression. Alice's disdain for allopathic medicine nearly cost her her life. Suicide is a frightening and very real possibility in depression. Fortunately, Alice was rescued by the helicopter of Imipramine before her bias against allopathic medicine led her to the Pearly Gates. Unfortunately, most of the alternative practitioners that Alice visited were not well informed about depression and failed to diagnose her problem. Since Alice had no medical partner she could trust, she was alone in traversing the maze of potential healing treatments that becomes more varied year by year.

Dr. David Eisenberg and his colleagues at Harvard Medical School published an article about Americans' use of alternative medical treatments that was featured in the January, 1993 volume of the *New England Journal of Medicine*. They questioned a random sample of 1,539 adults concerning their use of 16 diverse types of alternative treatments ranging from acupuncture and homeopathy to mental imagery and massage therapy. Thirty-four percent of the sample had used one or more of these treatment modalities in the previous year. Based on these data, the researchers estimated that Americans made approximately 425 million visits to alternative practitioners in 1990, compared to 338 million visits to allopathic primary care providers. Of the $13.7 billion spent on these alternative treatments, consumers paid $10.3 billion out of their own pockets. This sum exceeded the total amount that insurance companies paid for all hospitalizations in that year!

Era 1 medicine has typically looked upon alternative practices with a jaundiced eye. Although homeopathy is regarded as mainstream medicine throughout Europe, it is still regarded as an alternative—and perhaps a dangerous one at that—by the American medical establishment. The primary fear of most physicians is that a person will give up a potentially curative or life-enhancing Era 1 treatment in favor of an unproven, even harmful, remedy. In Alice's case, they might have been correct. Several studies have revealed, however, that the typical consumer of alternative medicine avoids the rigid stance of either Alice or the type of Christian Scientist that shuns Era 1 medicine entirely.

The profile of the average consumer of alternative healing services ought to come as a relief to physicians. The stereotype of the ill-informed, desperate patient ripe for conning by slick-talking snake-oil salesmen has not held up in studies. Research indicates that the typical consumer of alternative health care is above average in education and intent on choosing from among the most effective healing techniques. Such individuals are not attempting to avoid Era 1 medicine, but to educate themselves as to when it is best used by itself, not at all, or in combination with other therapies. For this reason, Miron and I agree with many of our colleagues that healing practices outside of the purview of Era 1 medicine are best called complementary therapies rather than alternative therapies. The best approach to healing is often "both and" rather than "either or."

Choices in cancer treatment are among the most difficult to make for the patient and of most concern to oncologists who help care for them. Michael Lerner is President of the Commonweal Foundation in Bolinas, California. After his father, journalist Max Lerner, was diagnosed with prostate cancer, Michael traveled around the world exploring complementary methods for cancer treatment. In the company of physician and yoga therapist Dr. Sandra McClanahan, Lerner toured facilities ranging from European medical centers offering more intensive chemotherapy than is available in the U.S., to the Laetrile clinics that dot the Mexican border. His extensive and meticulous research unearthed no miracle cures, although each center had its share of stunning testimonials.

Michael did find that those facilities that helped bring forth the intrinsic wholeness within a patient—through diet, exercise, meditation, and attention to the issues of healing one's life—certainly improved the quality of life. Although such centers generally keep no research data, perhaps the length of life was also increased in some cases. In the decade since Michael began his research, he has investigated cancer treatments throughout North America, India, Japan, and Europe. Drawing on the best of what he found, Michael and physician Rachel Naomi Remen founded the acclaimed Commonweal Cancer Help Program, a week-long residential healing retreat for those with cancer and their support persons. This program was featured in Bill Moyers' 1993 PBS documentary, *Healing and the Mind*.

Lerner's tremendous knowledge made him the perfect candidate to serve as a Special Consultant to the Office of Technology Assessment of the U.S. Congress from 1988 to 1990, as this office conducted a meticulous study entitled *Unconventional Cancer Treatments*. In 1994, Michael published the finest book available in the area of choices for cancer treatment. *Choices in Healing: Integrating the Best of Conventional and Complementary Approaches to Cancer* is a beacon of compassion and objectivity, hope, and good advice that encompasses the best in the physical, emotional, and spiritual healing that cancer invites one to experience.

In June of 1992, an official Office of Alternative Medicine was created within the National Institutes of Health. Although start-up funding for this office was a mere two million dollars, by June of 1993, 30 small research grants had been given out for projects such as the effects of:

- Qi Gong on reflex sympathetic dystrophy,
- tai chi on balance disorders,
- yoga on obsessive-compulsive disorder and heroin addiction,
- biofeedback training on diabetes,
- Ayurveda on Parkinson's disease,
- guided imagery on asthma,
- hypnosis on chronic pain,
- massage on bone marrow transplants,
- macrobiotic diet on cancer, and
- intercessory (when other individuals intervene on your behalf) prayer.

Alternative forms of medicine encompass all three eras of medicine. Whether they involve high-dose chemotherapy, prayer, energy medicine, or mental imagery, research is important. Our motto is, and has always been, "Keep an open mind, but don't let your brain fall out."

CHAPTER TEN

BODY AND SOUL:
Who Are We and Why Do We Get Sick?

Jeannie was a 32-year-old mother of twin 3-year-old daughters when she was diagnosed with inflammatory breast cancer. One of the most optimistic, hopeful people I've ever met, she taught me a lot about seeking out the best care for the body while honoring the needs of the soul.

Despite aggressive chemotherapy, a stringent macrobiotic diet, acupuncture treatment, regular yoga and meditation practice, tremendous support, and a great deal of prayer, Jeannie's cancer spread like wildfire. She is one of the many bright, loving people we know who are important reminders that when our time comes to die—no matter how loving, supported, and emotionally healed we are—our physical vehicles will return to dust so that our souls can be born once again. Jeannie's deep conviction that her physical body was only the house for her soul allowed her to approach death with a peaceful wisdom beyond her years.

Jeannie wrote each of her children a letter to be opened every year on their birthday, an idea that had originated with one of the first cancer patients I ever had the chance to work with. As I read some of the letters, I had the uncanny feeling that she actually knew her daughters at each age, and truly understood their hopes and fears. The letters carried with them the certainty that Jeannie would continue to be there for her children long after her body had passed away. She also taped stories for them about her own childhood and the challenges of growing up. She spoke of her parents and what she'd learned from them, about marrying their father, and how excited everyone had been at their births. She spoke, too, about her struggle with cancer and the tremendous grief she felt when she knew she'd have to leave them. She would miss their ball games and dances, their sore throats and report cards, their first periods, their weddings and the birth of their children. But, if her children remembered her, she promised she would be there in spirit for them.

An old Hasidic tale tells how the angels weep when a soul enters a physical body at birth and how they rejoice when it returns to the heavenly realms at death. This is a very different way of looking at life, isn't it? We usually think of our lives as straight lines beginning with birth and ending at death—the longer the line the better. In Native American tradition, in contrast, life is thought of as a circle. Whether the circle is small or large, death marks its completion rather than its destruction. Patients such as Jeannie helped me see death as part of the wholeness of life. Her death might have seemed premature to others, but *she* was able to see her life as complete.

Because Western culture worships youth and fitness, stories like Jeannie's may seem troublesome. She was so positive, so healed. Why did she become ill, and why did she die? There is an ancient story that I always think of when I ask myself those questions:

> *Before* Siddharta Gautama became the Buddha, he was a young prince supplied with every conceivable luxury. His father had gone to great lengths to keep him inside the palace, protected from exposure to suffering. One day the curious prince demanded that his charioteer take him into the city. Spying a sick person, he inquired, "What is that?" His charioteer explained that all human flesh was

heir to illness. Next he asked about a very old man, hobbling with a cane. Once again, the charioteer explained that all flesh had to age. Finally, Siddharta saw a corpse burning on a funeral pyre. Stunned, he asked whether that would happen to him and his family as well. Once again, the charioteer pointed out the impermanence of the human body.

The future Buddha was so distressed that he left the palace and took up the life of a renunciate holy man, vowing to find an end to suffering. The method that the Buddha eventually taught, following his enlightenment, did not obliterate sickness, old age, or death. Neither was it about using the power of your mind to manifest wealth or to win friends and influence people. Liberation was not about the body or about filling our endless desires. It was about attaining a state of peace, joy, wisdom, and compassion that was not dependent on any outside condition.

The Buddha's message is as powerful today as it was 2,500 years ago. But we have to have the ears to hear it. Perhaps the saddest misunderstanding of the power of the mind to heal is the twisting of the Buddha's message. Rather than transcending suffering, which means that we must learn and grow from it, the "New Age" message is that we can eliminate it. Just think right and you can cure illness, prevent aging, and possibly even live in your current body for hundreds of years, some New Agers offer. Perhaps at death you can even ascend, leaving a little pile of hair and fingernails. A few mystics have done just that, but by far, the greater majority have died of cancer and other diseases, often at young ages. Can we reasonably assume that these great masters were psychological basket cases or spiritual failures? The Buddha himself died of food poisoning, but not before explaining to the cook that his time here was done and he needed a doorway out of his body!

I once spoke at a health-care conference with several notable experts on body/mind and spirit. One of them tried to convince the audience that spiritual awakening is a sure-fire cure for illness. I could feel my blood start to boil as he went on and on about spirituality and perfect health.

Although a somewhat shy person, I stood up and challenged the speaker who, to me, represented a subtle, dangerous type of New Age Gestapo member. I explained that he was unleashing terror on people, giving them the impression that illness is—if not the result of the wages of sin—at least the badge of the unenlightened. I pointed out that all the mystics and spiritual teachers were dead, many of cancer. Upon hearing this protestation, the entire audience sprang to their feet and gave me a standing ovation! When the conference was over, the speaker I had challenged sought out Miron and me. His last attempt to uphold his dangerous thesis was that perhaps the saints I had cited really weren't enlightened after all!

You see, when we make perfect bodies the focus of our lives, we will inevitably be very disappointed. While we need to do what we can both to stay well and to cure our illnesses when possible, a total healing is not always our destiny. Miron and I have heard dozens of accounts of people's near-death experiences (NDE's) that speak to the question, "Why does illness occur?" One woman told us that during her NDE following a serious car crash, the Great Being of Light had offered her three choices: continue into the Light, return to earth with minor injuries, or return in a vegetative state. I was shocked by the last choice, but the woman explained that it wouldn't have been a hard choice to make had it been the right choice. After all, while on the Other Side, our earthly lives seem as short as a dream. The Being of Light showed this woman a life review of all the people she loved, with and without her being in a vegetative state. When it was clear that the vegetative state would not have occasioned any particular growth for anyone, she chose to return with minor injuries.

Betty Eadie, in her best-selling book, *Embraced by the Light*, recounts a fascinating insight that the Being of Light gave her. At one point, the heavens seemed to scroll back, and she was able to look down at the earth. She saw a homeless man and instantly "knew" that he had chosen this particular role in order to teach compassion to the wealthy psychiatrist whose office was down the block. Too often we've been taught to think that poverty or illness is a divine punishment, or at least our "bad karma" returning to us! Perhaps, as Betty Eadie and countless others have experienced, some life events are actually soul contracts that we agreed to for our own or someone else's benefit. That puts an entirely different twist on the question of why a beautiful, caring young mother such as Jeannie would get sick, doesn't it?

Think about Jeannie's story for a moment. Now, think about someone you know who died young or who had or has a serious illness. Can you imagine that their illness may in fact be a gift, an act of service, that helps other people toward a more compassionate awareness?

Physician Raymond Moody was one of the first people to write about the NDE. When his classic book, *Life after Life*, was published in 1978, very few people had even heard of NDE's, although reports of such events exist in the literature of every culture. In the years that have passed since Moody brought the phenomenon to public attention, the term *near-death experience* has become a household phrase.

With the publication of *Heading Toward Omega: The Meaning of the Near-Death Experience*, psychologist Kenneth Ring ushered in a scientific era in the study of mystical states. Ring's detailed questionnaires allowed him to map several phases of the NDE. Not every person experiences each phase, but a small percentage report having an entire, or *core*, near-death experience. The first phase is marked by a transcendent feeling of peace. The only words I can summon to describe my own experience of this phenomenon comprise the biblical phrase, "The peace that passeth understanding." The person then has the feeling of lifting up out of their body. Some people experience leaving through a hole in the top of their head, a location that corresponds to the crown, or seventh chakra, of the energy body.

People often comment that looking down at their bodies from a perspective that we are totally unused to is most unnerving. In fact, it is sometimes hard to recognize the body beneath them as their own. Rather than feeling bad about their dying body, most people report a curious detachment from it. We have heard it described as the husk of a seed that has sprouted or the clothes taken off at the end of the day. People at this stage often describe scenes of physicians attempting to resuscitate them. They may also have a thought of family, for example, and find themselves instantly in another locale, observing the person they were thinking about. Remarkably, it's not that unusual for a family member to see the apparition of a dying loved one as it makes its final rounds.

The next phase of the NDE is marked by very rapid movement. The most common description is that of hurtling through a dark tunnel. Sometime during this process, other beings who may be described as dead relatives, angels, helpers, or guides arrive to assist the soul in its journey.

At the end of the tunnel comes a meeting with a Divine Light that emanates perfect love and deep acceptance. This Light is alternately described as God, Jesus, an angel, or a Supreme Being of Light. The experience of Divine Light, which I have been graced with on four separate occasions, is inexplicable. We simply have no words for it. To say the experience is pure love, absolute forgiveness, and incomprehensible wisdom is a very pale facsimile. Most people who have this experience simply don't want it to end. It is the most beautiful, blissful state imaginable. People leave it very grudgingly, either because they are informed at this point that it isn't yet time for them to die, or because they are given a choice about whether to continue further into the experience or return to their bodies.

Almost everyone we've ever talked to about their NDE said that they did not want to return to life on earth. It's too hard here, too far from the love that our soul recognizes as home. Nonetheless, people who make the choice to return usually do so for one of two reasons. The most common is a commitment to raising their children. The second is a strong knowing that their life has a specific purpose that has not yet been fulfilled.

A friend of ours who had tried to commit suicide as a teenager was not given a choice, but a reprimand. She was told that life was sacred, a great opportunity, and to take this life was to deny our part in God's plan. When she complained bitterly that no one loved her, listing the shortcomings of her parents, the Being of Light told her with great tenderness that she would have to learn to love herself, that she could never feel the love of another person until she truly loved herself.

Shortly after we heard about this incident, we met another woman who had been so abused that she had tried to kill herself at the age of seven by sledding downhill headfirst into a cement bench. Her experience was similar—she was told quite sternly, and yet with total love, to return to her body and to learn to love herself.

People who have NDE's that result from suicides rarely try to take their lives again. Often, they become explicitly aware of the value of all the trials, obstacles, and even horrors of their lives— how every trauma and disappointment had the potential of contributing to their (or other people's) wisdom and capacity to love. They've gotten the message that life is a privilege.

The Buddhists say that if there was an ocean the size of the Universe, with a wooden hoop floating on its surface, getting a human birth would be about as likely as a lone turtle swimming in that endless sea, sticking his head up through the wooden ring. It may seem trite, but life really is a gift and a privilege.

Interestingly enough, about a third of all people who have an NDE also experience a life review. However, this life review does not consist of the familiar sense of one's life rushing in front of one's eyes that some people describe when they have a brush with death (but don't actually leave their bodies). Instead, the Supreme Being of Light conducts the review, during which all of life seems to appear at once, like a hologram. Rather than reviewing the events of life through one's own eyes, the review consists of evaluating one's relationships through the eyes of the people you actually related to. If you caused pain for another person, you feel that pain. If you brought joy or encouragement to someone, you feel that, too.

Many people have told us that the life review was the most difficult experience they have ever had, and also the most important. We are ultimately responsible for all our actions. The problem is not one of God forgiving us. As one woman said, that's a given. The real question is, can you forgive yourself when you understand the depths of your own lovelessness. Time and time again, we've been told that the lesson of the NDE is one of love. We take human birth in order to learn about giving and receiving love, and in the process, we become wiser and more creative. We are like growing edges of the Divine Mind, developing the love and wisdom to become part of the co-creative process through which the Universe expands.

Some Christian fundamentalists once presented us with a magazine that described how Satan was responsible for the NDE. After all, the article reasoned, Lucifer is a fallen angel whose name means *light*. The article stated that the devil is trying to trick us into believing that we are loved in spite of our mistakes. If we believe him, we may slack off in our efforts to improve ourselves, and fare poorly on Judgment Day.

I tried to explain to these fundamentalists that Jesus had specified how we could evaluate the truth of various teachers and experiences. He told us to look at their results—"by their fruits ye shall know them." Psychologist Kenneth Ring has researched the effects that NDE's have on people, and their fruits are very good indeed. People who have NDE's do believe that God has forgiven them for their ignorant actions, but that doesn't mean that they become apathetic when it comes to displaying human kindness. In fact, compassion and responsibility are much enhanced.

There have been several reports concerning hardened criminals who had NDE's and were instantly reformed, more interested in helping others than in serving their own needs. Whether you believe in Satan or not, how can such a positive change be the result of anything evil? How can we go wrong with respect, benevolence, and the urge to listen for the voice of God—doing the Divine will rather than our own?

People whose NDE's continue beyond the life review are sometimes given a mini-tour of the Other Side. What they see is varied. Many have reported "lost souls" drifting through a gray mist. These souls apparently do not know that they are dead. A woman we met who had an NDE as a child asked the Being of Light about these souls. He pointed out that there were angels all around them, and if they asked for help, the angels would take them to the Light. Help could not be given unless asked for, however, since human beings have free will.

Another woman reported seeing people in various "hell states." These hells, she realized, were projections of their own fears. As soon as they either recognized that, or asked for aid, they could move on. This latter experience is very reminiscent of Tibetan Buddhist teachings on the *bardo states*.

According to this philosophy, after we have gone through the light experience, the soul then proceeds through a variety of intermediate (bardo) states between death and rebirth, either on earth or in some other realm. As we move through these bardos, we are met with the projections of our own minds. In one bardo that seems like an apt description of a fundamentalist hell, our fears seem like wrathful deities (devils) attacking us. Our doubts assault us. Our ignorance returns to us. At any stage we can "wake up" and find ourselves back in the Light. Should we do that, we realize the true power of our minds to heal.

Once awakened to the true power of the mind, we are "enlightened," awakened to who we really are. We can then apparently choose to come back to earth to help others or continue on into other realms. In the Tibetan tradition, the homeless man of whom Betty Eadie spoke would be recognized as a *Bodhisattva*, a person who returns not because of his own needs, but to help others. The angels cry as much at the birth of a Bodhisattva as they do for the rest of us. Every soul, no matter how enlightened, forgets the Love from which it springs in order to play its role here on earth.

CHAPTER ELEVEN

ILLNESS AND PARADIGM SHIFTS

Before the 14th century, the reigning paradigm, or belief system, about health and illness involved our relationship with God. If we led an exemplary life, we were supposed to be rewarded with good health. Then, during the 14th century, the black plague swept across Europe, eventually killing one-third of the population.

The Catholic Church was quick to look for a scapegoat. At first they blamed the Jews for poisoning the wells, even though the Jews were dying just like everyone else. In village after village, supposedly religious people tortured innocent Jews in the name of God, wresting false confessions from them and then burning them to death. Still, the plague continued. The Church then turned to another scapegoat—witches. Between the 14th and 17th centuries, anywhere from half a million to as many as nine million women were brutally tortured until they confessed that they were witches. Still, the plague continued. Eventually, Europeans concluded that staying on God's right side wasn't an adequate health-insurance program. They looked to science instead.

Sadly, many of us are still stuck in the mindset of the medieval Church. If we could just do things right, some of us think, then God will reward us. The New Age twist on this same old notion is that if we are good people, we will have good karma and we won't get sick. Therefore, karmic fundamentalists—like religious fundamentalists—may reason that any misfortune must be evidence of previous wrongdoing.

Science may be able to cure our bodies at times, but it cannot cure thinking that is steeped in the illusion that a small-minded God punishes His creation with illness, either directly or through bad karma. The cure for this kind of thinking lies neither in religion nor in science, but in a paradigm shift—an awakening out of the dreams of fear into the reality of Divine Love. In my book, *Fire in the Soul*, I called this awakening a shift to spiritual optimism. This concept brings to mind the time that Albert Einstein was asked what the most important question was that a human being needed to answer. He responded, "Is the universe a friendly place or not?"

Oftentimes, we're too busy making a living and raising the kids to even think about Einstein's response. Illness, however, puts us face to face with our beliefs and stimulates thinking about life's most important questions. Illness brings about the need to create meaning from tragedy—to reinvent our lives on a higher, wiser, more loving level than before.

In 1977, Belgian physicist Ilya Prigogine won a Nobel prize for his Theory of Dissipative Structures—a kind of chaos theory. He showed that a period of dissolution is required before any system—whether a society, a solar system, or a molecule—can jump to a higher level of organization. His discovery solved an apparent paradox.

The Second Law of Thermodynamics states that everything in the universe is in a state of decay, yet more complex structures are nonetheless evolving. It seems that everything from the stock market to the evolution of the species proceeds in a very disorderly manner, contrary to the ordered progression that our old scientific paradigm predicted. This nonlinearity (disorderly evolution) is coupled with interdependence (communication and feedback between different parts of the system). Nonlinearity and interdependence together create chaos, which has been defined as "unpredictability without randomness." You can read more about this intriguing field in *Chaos and the Evolving Ecological Universe*, by Sally Goerner.

The physical principles that Prigogine discovered dash any hope of being in control and thus assuring the outcome of the events in our lives. On the other hand, they allow for a Mystery that orchestrates those events and assures that the threads of what may appear to be disaster and random error are eventually incorporated into the Wholeness of an unseen tapestry. Prigogine quotes the writer Vladimir Nabokov, "What is real cannot be controlled; what can be controlled is not real."

Seen through the lens of chaos theory, the disintegration of the former Soviet Union is a creative event because it makes room for newness and growth. If you've read Kahlil Gibran's classic work, *The Prophet*, you may remember that he expressed a similar sentiment through poetry, which, like mathematics, is a language of the soul. "Pain," said Gibran, "is the bitter pill of the inner physician that cracks the shell of our understanding." A seed can only grow into a flower when it has swelled and died. Likewise, our own ability to create newness in our lives comes from periods of crisis that force us to put our old behaviors and beliefs to rest.

What kinds of stories do you tell yourself when illness or some other difficult situation crops up? Stop for a moment and think about some unpleasant event that happened to you—what was the story you told yourself about why it happened?

If your story had to do with growth, love, or understanding, then you can probably reflect upon periods of crisis and realize that they were important times of change even though you would not have imagined or chosen the series of chaotic events that led you to a new perspective. If your story was negative and fearful, you probably feel or felt helpless and disempowered. If we believe that we are helpless victims of other people, or recipients of God's righteous anger, how else are we going to feel?

Psychologists actually classify people as optimists or pessimists by the stories they tell themselves about why bad things happen. Pessimists usually offer three types of mental explanations that researcher Martin Seligman from the University of Pennsylvania sums up as "It's all my fault. I mess up everything I do, and it's the story of my life." This kind of reasoning is called internal because you blame yourself, global because you think you are a failure across the board, and stable because you think that misfortune is the story of your life. After all, if you believe you're stupid today, it's unlikely you'll get smart tomorrow.

Optimists, on the other hand, reveal the stress-hardy attitudes first described by psychologist Suzanne Kobasa when she studied a company that was undergoing divestiture. Some people thrived in the chaos, while others couldn't tolerate uncertainty and began to show both the physical and emotional toll of stress. The hardy people were described as "transformational" copers. Rather than trying to return the situation to its status quo, which is called *regressive coping*, they were ready for changes. Their readiness translated into the three characteristic attitudes: challenge, commitment, and control. They viewed change and chaos as a challenge. They felt a commitment to some kind of goal or higher vision that presented an expanded frame of reference through which to view the current problem, and they felt in control of themselves even though the situation might have been uncontrollable.

During the seven years that I directed the Mind/Body clinic at Boston's Beth Israel and New England Deaconess hospitals, I had the chance to hear hundreds of people's optimistic and pessimistic stories about why bad things had happened to them. And, although, as you know, we don't subscribe to a one-to-one correspondence between thinking and health, I observed first-hand that those stories certainly did have some effect on the course of illness. At times, that effect was tremendous, leading to very rapid death on the one hand, or unexpected remission on the other. Most people came to the clinic at a point in their lives when illness had presented a new and sometimes overwhelming challenge. As I heard their stories, I became much more aware of my own. While the mind/body program was based on using meditation to bring forth what our director Herbert Benson called the relaxation response, perhaps the most important thing our patients learned was to release the regrets and resentments that formed the foundation for pessimistic stories. We will be doing some of this work together in Chapters 18 and 19.

When individuals entered the Mind/Body Clinic, they were given a battery of psychological questionnaires so that we could assess how they felt at the outset, and then measure changes in attitude both right after the program and six months later. One of the questions asked was whether these people felt that they were being, or should be, punished for their sins. When I discovered that a majority of people actually answered yes to that question, I was stunned.

We were offering an excellent program, the purpose being to reduce people's stress, but we had left out the most basic question of all—our relationship to the Universe. After all, what good is a course in meditation and diaphragmatic breathing, mindfulness, and exercise if you are telling yourself stories about a God who is some kind of cosmic peeping Tom, a God with a little black book full of your sins and shortcomings that "He" will tally up to decide whether you deserve reward or punishment? On the flip side, the story that says that the Universe is meaningless and events are random, is stressful as well.

I once appeared on a radio talk show, discussing the fact that stress is a result of feeling separate, and that separateness is the result of fear. One unfortunate man called in to say that his greatest fear was going to hell. I asked if he'd committed a crime that he had not confessed and made amends for. He said no, that on the contrary, he was a very moral person, always trying to do good for others. But, he added, God is omniscient and sees all our thoughts. Since he sometimes had thoughts of anger, lust, or jealousy he believed that on Judgment Day he would be thrown into hell for eternity. As you might imagine, this man was a walking study in stress-related disorders. Is it any wonder? Worse still, he viewed his symptoms as evidence that he was already being punished by God.

When I asked this man if anyone went to heaven, he was silent for a moment. Finally, he offered hesitantly, "Maybe Mother Teresa." It was obvious that this man was not only a psychological pessimist who blamed himself for the problems in his life, but he was also a religious pessimist, a person who not only believes that he is bad, but also that God will no doubt punish him for it. I often cite a study of a hundred Catholics that links religious beliefs to self-esteem. Unquestionably, the study could also have been done of a hundred Jews or a hundred Protestants. The researchers chose one religious group simply because they had all learned the same dogma. They found that the higher people's self-esteem was, the more likely they were to view God as loving and merciful. The lower the level of self-esteem, the more likely they were to view God as punitive. Self-esteem is related to how we were raised. If our parents were loving, self-esteem is likely to be high; if they were punitive and authoritarian, it is likely to be low. It seems that the stories we tell ourselves about God are simply continuations of the images we have about our parents.

In *Guilt Is the Teacher, Love Is the Lesson,* I help the reader consider and heal old religious beliefs and the psychological wounds upon which they are based. When people become ill, this is often the kind of healing that is most pressing. When we're diagnosed with multiple sclerosis, AIDS, or any life-challenging illness, we don't know where we stand. Life as we have known it crumbles. Who we were dies, and we have not yet been reborn to who we will be. This period of uncertainty is a sacred time, but also a vulnerable period in which all our beliefs come up for reconsideration.

The 15th-century Christian mystic, St. John of the Cross, coined the term *dark night of the soul* to describe this passage. The dark night, he believed, was an indispensable part of the spiritual journey, as it is precisely during these chaotic times when the greatest potential for breakthrough and healing exist. Essentially, at such times we are forced to shift our paradigm—to give up our old way of being and explore a new room in our life.

Perhaps you know the parable of the college professor and the Buddhist monk. The professor had heard of the monk's great wisdom and decided to pay him a visit. They sat at a table opposite one another, and the monk began to pour tea. He filled the cup and kept right on pouring until tea had covered the table! The professor jumped up in alarm, but the monk just smiled and said, "Your mind is like this teacup. It is already so full that no more can fit in."

Crisis and illness can empty our cups in a hurry. Oftentimes, though, we need help to decide on how best to refill them. All too often, our religious priesthood is as out of touch with sources of wisdom as is our secular priesthood, therapists, and psychiatrists, who may think more in terms of pathology than they do of growth and potential. Many hospitals, however, do have excellent pastoral counseling departments to help people through their dark nights. A study by Drs. Elisabeth McSherry and William Nelson at a Veteran's Administration Hospital in Massachusetts reviewed the effects of daily visits by trained pastoral counselors on recuperation from surgery. They found that the total length of stay was reduced by 27 percent, calls for nursing help by 33 percent, and use of pain medication by 33 percent. Just sharing our feelings about our crises can help us heal faster because we no longer feel we are alone.

We can learn a great deal about shifting the paradigm of illness and crisis by observing how more "primitive" societies treat people in transition. Anthropologist Victor Turner is well known for his study of the ritual process in different cultures. A ritual is a rite of passage, a transition between two distinct states of being or stations in society. The traditional rite of passage consists of three distinct stages: the *separation* from one's previous state of being; the *liminal period,* during which one dwells between two worlds—not-here not-there—and the *reincorporation* into some new role or status in the society. The ambiguous, intermediate state of liminality—of dwelling at the threshold of a new life—is often compared to being in the womb, in a state of darkness and invisibility or wandering in the wilderness.

The Jews wandered in the wilderness for 40 years when they left bondage in Egypt before they were reborn to a new life in Palestine. Jesus wandered in the wilderness for 40 days after his baptism, which was also a rite of passage. During that time he deeply considered his beliefs. Would he serve his fears (which in the pictorial language of the unconscious appears as Satan), or would he serve the unknown God? This is the question that darkness calls up for each of us.

The collective hypnosis, our unconscious adherence to the familiar beliefs that guide our life, is broken in the liminal period when we are offered up to the threshold of the unknown. During times of transition, we awaken from the familiar trance of life and find ourselves in alien territory. If we knew that this frightening, unknown period was a necessary transition, such as the transition period of labor, we could more easily ask for whatever help was needed and more patiently hold on and wait for the birth. We could take comfort in the fact that the process is natural, not pathological.

Each dark night and little death challenges us to re-evaluate our paradigm. What a difference it would make if a person in the throes of a life crisis were called an initiate—and then skillfully led to a rebirth. Part of the value of suffering is that it initiates or intensifies the search for what is most sacred, for only in placing our minds on a higher vision can we emerge from the liminal period—not only intact, but healed.

A Navajo legend compares human life to a beautifully woven rug. When seen from the bottom, the earth side, the rug seems to be made of random patterns and loose ends. But when seen from above, the spiritual side, all the dark threads and zigzags are an integral part of the magnificent pattern.

PART TWO

The Art and Practices of Healing

CHAPTER TWELVE

REFRAMING:
The Art of Making a Paradigm Shift

Miron loves to tell the story about a frequent traveler from Chicago who had searched for a house in a quiet neighborhood with easy access to O'Hare Airport. He loved living there until a new runway was constructed, placing his home directly beneath the flight path of incoming planes. The planes flew so low that he could actually see people in the windows. The noise and lack of privacy were driving him crazy. Feeling increasingly anxious and stressed, he consulted a psychologist, who took him through a problem-solving session. When it was clear that he couldn't move because no one would want his house and that the external situation wouldn't change, the psychologist suggested that he would have to change his mind. Easy for someone else to say, isn't it?

A year passed, and one day the psychologist happened to run into the man at a shopping mall. When he asked his former client about his problem, the man smiled like the cat who's just lapped up some half-and-half. He'd taken the psychologist's advice and changed his mind by putting his problem in a new frame of reference. One night when the sound of the planes was making him furious, an idea suddenly popped into his head. The next day he went to the hardware store and bought a big bucket of white paint. He climbed up on his roof and in huge block letters printed "Welcome to Cleveland." Now when he hears a plane overhead, he bursts out laughing instead of cursing.

Some of the greatest healers are capable of helping us make similar changes in perception. Milton Ericson is a noted healer who was the most famous medical hypnotist of all times. Hypnosis, of course, is the creation of a particular frame of reference. Ericson was a psychiatrist who learned his craft partly through a life crisis when polio left him paralyzed as an adolescent. One day Ericson's parents left him alone, strapped into a chair. Bored and wishing that he could get to the window, he began to fantasize about walking over to it. As he used his imagination, muscles that had been paralyzed began to twitch. Before long, Ericson had learned to use his imagination to coordinate groups of muscles and rehabilitate himself! During his long convalescence, he became a keen observer of the power of the imagination—of mindset and frame of reference.

Since Ericson lived on a farm, he had ample opportunity to observe animal behavior. One day when his father couldn't get a balky cow into the barn, Ericson suggested that he grab hold of her tail and pull backwards. The cow, of course, resisted and walked straight into the barn! Our minds can be as contrary, and also as easy to change, as the cow's. Ericson often told his patients stories that instantly changed their frame of reference and subsequently affected both attitude and health.

For example, one of his patients was a little girl with so many freckles that she felt disfigured. She didn't want to go to school anymore and became withdrawn and depressed. When her mother brought her to Ericson, he stood with his hands on his hips and bellowed at her like a bull, "You're a thief. I know you're a thief." Well, this really confounded her mindset. She was quaking in her boots, trying to figure out what she'd stolen. She certainly wasn't thinking about her freckles.

By surprising her, Ericson had created an altered state of reality that is called an *indirect induction* of hypnosis. Once her attention was anchored in this receptive state, he told the child an elaborate story of how he had seen her sneaking into the kitchen, taking out a ladder, and reaching into the cookie jar on top of the refrigerator. When she finally realized that he was making up a story and she was off the hook as a thief, relief flooded through her body. At just that moment, Ericson got to the punchline; the jar full of cookies fell down and the cinnamon splattered all over the little girl's face. That, he laughed, was how she got her freckles. From that moment on, freckles brought forth the feelings of relief and delight that Ericson had induced, and her anxiety was gone. The freckles now inhabited another frame of reference!

Miron and I never met Milton Ericson, but we have met other healers who work in a similar way. For many years, we did research in psychoneuroimmunology with psychologist David McClelland, who was then a professor at Harvard. Dave is well known for his studies of human motivation—the need for power, the need for achievement, the need for friendship, and the like. He also has an avid interest in healers and healing and had conducted preliminary research on a local healer in Cambridge, Massachusetts. At the first sign of cold symptoms, he had Harvard students report either to the health service or to Karmu, the healer.

Karmu's patients fared better than those assigned to the health service. They reported less severe symptoms and fewer days lost from school. Furthermore, some of them recovered immediately and completely after their visit to Karmu. Miron was intrigued and asked Dave how he thought Karmu healed people. Dave just laughed and said, "He messes with your mind."

Several months later, Miron had a chance to experience that mind-messing on a first-hand basis. He was hard at work, in the middle of a huge experiment. His laboratory was hopping with lab technicians, graduate students, and postdoctoral fellows all feverishly working because it was time to submit a grant renewal for their research. Mid-morning Miron started to feel sick. His sinuses filled up, and he was overtaken by body aches and fatigue. Finding it increasingly difficult to concentrate, he decided to go home and lie in bed, drinking fluids and taking aspirin for a day or two while he supervised the experiment by phone.

Dejected about this state of affairs, he got into his car and started to drive home when, suddenly, Karmu popped into his mind. He knew exactly where Karmu lived, so he drove over there and rang the bell. No one answered, so he went up the stairs to the apartment. The door was open, and the entrance smelled warm and inviting since there was a big pot of soup cooking on the kitchen stove. He knocked, but there was no answer. Finally, he stepped in and called out. A resonant voice came from the back of the house, welcoming him in.

Miron walked down a long hall into a bedroom where the TV was blaring loudly. There on the bed was a mountain of a black man sitting in his underwear and drinking port wine from a bottle. Miron asked in amazement, "Are you Karmu?"

The very engaging and mischievous healer smiled beatifically and began to kid him. "Are you a movie star? You're so good-looking. Come on, now, I'm sure I've seen you in the movies." And when Karmu had Miron as totally confused and disarmed as Ericson's freckled patient, he asked what was wrong.

"Well, Karmu," Miron stammered, "I'm a friend of Professor McClelland's from Harvard. He told me that you could cure colds, and since I have one coming on, I was wondering if you could help me."

The mysterious Karmu beckoned Miron to approach him, reaching under his bed and producing a jar of putrid-looking purple liquid. "Purple medicine," he announced. Miron paled at the thought of drinking this brew, but Karmu motioned him over to the bureau to get a glass and gave him clear instructions. "Fill the glass up full, and then go down the hall and run the tub one-third full of lukewarm water. Pour in the purple medicine, and then sit in it for exactly 11 minutes."

Miron dutifully walked down the hall, feeling that he was past the point of no return. He began to laugh at the thought of what our colleagues would think if they could see him now. He stripped off his clothes, ran the tub, and sat in the sea of purple water, timing himself for exactly 11 minutes. The longer he sat, the funnier it seemed. Finally finished, he stood up to get out and dry himself, only to find that he was purple from the waist down! And it would not rub off. He laughed even harder when he thought of the look I would have on my face that night when I saw him. He went back to Karmu's bedroom and was pronounced healed. Sure enough, when Miron got back into the car, he was feeling great. All of his symptoms had disappeared, and he was able to go back to work and finish his experiment.

What did Karmu do? It's simple. Just as Dave McClelland had said, Karmu had messed with Miron's mind. He confused him totally, turning a groaning pessimist into a laughing optimist.

Milton Ericson would have recognized Karmu as a master of indirect hypnosis. All of us are under hypnosis all the time, of course, because of our beliefs. The art of using the power of our minds to heal comes through the ability to *notice* when we are stuck in an unproductive mindset—to become *aware* of the mental movies that are limiting our creativity—and to make new choices. The two keys to inner healing are *awareness* and *choice*. With these keys, we can learn to awaken from the unconscious trance of life into a much more creative reality.

Miron and I once attended a Sunday service at a Church of Religious Science in Santa Monica, California. Agape (pronounced *ug-ah'-pay*, which means *compassionate love*), as the church is called, is a marvelous melting pot for black and white, Oriental and Hispanic peoples, and everyone else. The old warehouse that is home to Agape is filled to overflowing on Sunday mornings, when over 3,000 people show up at the two services. As Miron and I waited expectantly, ushers were still trying to seat people ten minutes after the service was scheduled to start. The emcee stood up and said simply that if we were upset by the commotion, we were cordially invited to change our minds. We all laughed, and immediately a sense of peace overcame me. My frame of reference shifted from impatience to an invitation to experience the peacefulness that is always available within.

After all, why should our peace of mind be dependent on external events? Psychiatrist Jerry Jampolsky, who has done so much to popularize *A Course in Miracles,* reminds us that we always have a choice in what we experience. Whenever I manage to work myself up into a good snit, I try to stop for a minute, take a deep breath, and remind myself of Jerry's words, "I could choose peace instead of this." It is extremely important to use these principles throughout the day—to remember the power of a deep breath coupled with a mental phrase that reminds you to let go and make a new choice.

Take a minute now *and think about a time today when your mind was controlling you and creating fear, anger, or frustration. Imagine yourself taking a breath and shifting your frame of reference. You might wish to try "I could choose peace instead of this," or to invent another frame of reference specific to your situation.*

In his classic book, *Varieties of Religious Experience*, the great physician and psychologist William James said, "I have no doubt whatever that most people live, whether physically, intellectually, or morally, in a very restricted circle of their potential being. They make use of a very small portion of their possible consciousness— much like a man who, out of his whole bodily organism, should get into a habit of using and moving only his little finger. We all have reservoirs of life to draw upon, of which we do not dream."

Miron and I traveled to Southern India in the spring of 1989 to participate in the First International Conference of Holistic Health and Medicine in Bangalore. While we were there, Miron had the opportunity to meet a holy man by the name of Sai Baba who knew how to draw upon the great reservoirs of life that William James was talking about. Although greatly revered in India, Sai Baba is a subject of controversy in the United States because he has a *siddhi*, or yogic mind power, that apparently enables him to manifest things out of thin air. A chubby man with long slim fingers, an infectious smile, and a surprising afro, Sai Baba often plucks gifts out of the air for his visitors.

Miron was sitting in a room with about 30 other participants from the conference when Sai Baba manifested a ring for the conference chairperson, Dr. Isaac Mathai. The ring fit perfectly, as we are told they always do. While Dr. Mathai was admiring the ring on his finger, Sai Baba touched it. The colorless stone changed instantly to a light green gem that glowed with a strange inner light. It was a very interesting demonstration of mental power that was calcu-lated to draw attention, but the alchemy that Sai Baba and other such masters are really interested in is the transformation of fear into love.

Books and tapes that tell you how to use your mind-power to manifest health, prosperity, and love are abundant and popular. There are also books that reveal how to use the power of your mind to seek revenge on your enemies and to curse those whom you judge. Power is a dangerous, two-edged sword. The truth is that most of us don't have nearly the mental power required to manifest anything at all, and that is most fortunate. If we had such power, think of the terrible harm we could do. Do you remember King Midas? His fervent desire was that everything he touched would turn to gold. After this wish was granted, he could no longer eat, drink, or hug a loved one because *everything* turned to gold. His greed destroyed everything that was most precious in life.

Did *you* ever wish for something and then realize how much better off you were without it? When I was an impoverished grad-uate student, Sandy, a teller at my bank, won a lottery with a big jackpot. Every week I made it a point to ask her how the money was changing her life. By the second week, Sandy was already wishing that she'd never won. The money had become a bone of contention among her husband, her parents, and her in-laws. Friends, relatives, and strangers were all fighting for a piece of it, and peace of mind had flown out the window. A year after she won the jackpot, Sandy was divorced. Manifesting a jackpot, or turning everything we touch into gold, may not be the best use of the full power of our minds.

Another potential pitfall to using mind power is the tremen-dous responsibility and consciousness that it entails. For example, did you ever wish someone dead when you got mad? Similarly, think of all the common expressions in our language: *I'm heart-sick. I'm dead tired. I'm as hungry as a horse.* So if you want to develop the power to manifest with your mind—to be a true co-creator with God—you'd better learn to overcome your fear, negativity, and unconsciousness first. The old yogis have always cautioned against spiritual materialism, the desire to develop powerful siddhis, because they can bring the practitioner into great danger. Although such powers tend to manifest as a natural part of spiritual development, real teachers counsel their students to ignore them rather than to court them.

Of course, if you're interested in using the power of your mind to improve your material situation, you probably can to some extent. But in addition to the dangers we have discussed, real siddhis don't come easily. It may take years of meditation, prayer, and intense inner work to accomplish what some best-selling books glibly promise with a few affirmations. But if you really want a prosperous life, there's an easier way to go about things. Jesus said it well when he taught his disciples to seek the Kingdom of Heaven first, and then all things would be added unto them.

If you seek peace and love first, if you learn to become mindfully present, you'll find that good things seem to be attracted to you without your even having to specify them. When you think about using the power of your mind in daily life, remember that peace is the most important goal, because thoughts of peace open the heart to love, and they close the mind to fear. Peace and love are the frame of reference through which we discover the mind's true power.

CHAPTER THIRTEEN

LETTING GO OF FEAR:
The Choice for Creativity and Love

Once upon a time there was a woman named Sheila who'd tried everything she could to overcome her fear and selfishness. She had been to therapy, attended dozens of workshops, and read countless books. As Sheila learned to pay closer attention to her thinking, she noticed that she was stuck in judgment a lot of the time. She judged her husband as lazy when he needed to rest. She judged her children for not trying harder in school. She relentlessly judged anyone who messed up the house, ate too much fat, or watched too many hours of television.

Sheila perceived her family as an extension of herself, and since she wanted to appear perfect, she needed them to seem perfect. Underneath the need for perfection, of course, was the fear of rejection. The fear of being judged by others, found unworthy, and abandoned is the basic terror that haunts the unconscious mind of all people. Sheila was aware of all of this and was at the stage of personal growth that Miron and I call being an "insightful neurotic."

Sick and tired of feeling stuck, Sheila decided to consult a wise woman who lived up on top of a mountain. The wise woman said, "Sheila, first thing when you get up in the morning, say to yourself, 'I am grateful for everything that happens, and I have no complaints at all.' During the day when you find yourself judging something, once again remind yourself, 'I am grateful for this, and I have no complaints at all.'"

Sheila went home and followed the wise woman's advice meticulously for an entire year. But at the end of the year, she still felt filled with self-criticism, fear, and judgment. Dejected after all of her efforts, Sheila returned to the wise woman and complained that the technique hadn't worked. Sheila still felt as self-centered as before. The wise woman looked into her eyes with a smile and said, "And I am grateful for this, and I have no complaints at all."

Needless to say, Sheila "got it" in that moment. We adapted Sheila's story from a Zen teaching tale of the poet and writer, Stephen Mitchell. The punchline of such stories always involves a paradigm shift, an "aha" when an intellectual insight becomes an essential knowing, and the person's world view is forever changed. Sheila's shift was out of the ego's fears of abandonment into the deep security of the Higher Self.

Did you ever see the movie *Defending Your Life*? It's about two people who have just died and who are reviewing their lives in a wild and wonderful place called Judgment City. In this place, you realized that the measure of your life was in whether or not you had learned to overcome fear. If you had succeeded, you progressed to the next step of evolution; otherwise, you had to reincarnate so you could try all over again.

We liked the film for two reasons. First, you got to eat whatever you wanted in Judgment City without gaining weight. Second, we do believe that the purpose of this life is in learning to transform fear into love.

In order to overcome fear, we need to acquaint ourselves with the wiles of the ego. The late Wolfgang Luther, a physician who founded an excellent body/mind healing practice called Autogenic Training, referred to the ego as "the dirty tricks department of the mind."

One of the ways in which the dirty tricks department works is through rumination. Everything might be okay now, but *"what if?" What if* are the two most loaded words in the English language. They can turn any situation into a catastrophe. I once had a lump in my breast that was suspicious enough that it needed to be removed. Not once did I ruminate on the thought, "What if it turns out to be nothing?" Instead, my mind ran around in circles "what iffing" about the possibility of it being cancer. What if it has spread? What if I die?

The "what ifs" led to questions about the meaning of the hypothetical cancer— which did, thankfully, turn out to be nothing at all, although I wore myself out with worry. Was this fantasized cancer an awakening experience? Was I about to undergo a spiritual transformation like so many people who grow as the result of their illness, or was it a meaningless event in a random universe? Have *you* ever run yourself ragged with a good case of the "what ifs"?

Back in those days, I was deeply engaged in reconsidering my most basic beliefs. It would have been wonderful if someone had presented me with a broader, less fearful, perspective on the "what ifs." That's just what I tried to do for the reader in *Fire in the Soul*, and we have adapted a *what if* exercise from that book for you. The best way to approach these "what ifs," which are basic reframes to heal the dirty tricks department of your mind—is to act as if they are a meditation. If you relax and focus on what is being said, the new images that arise in your body/mind can help cancel out some of the old fearful ones.

Please stop and try this exercise before reading on. Either tape the script below and play it back for yourself, or have someone read it to you slowly and thoughtfully. Pause at the dots so that the words have ample opportunity to reach deeply into your every cell. Be sure to do the exercise in a safe, comfortable place where you will not be disturbed. If possible, play some soft, inspiring music in the background, such as Pachelbel's Kanon in D *or the music of Bach.*

SHIFTING FROM FEAR TO LOVE

Take a deep breath...a big letting-go
breath...and when you're ready, allow
your eyes to close. Take a little
stretch...and get as comfortable as you

can. You might want to do a few head rolls or shoulder stretches, whatever would help you relax....

Now focus on your breathing. Take another big breath, and let it go completely....Now imagine that your belly is rising on the inbreath, letting go on the outbreath....Or you might feel like your whole body rises and falls with the tide of your breath....

You can deepen your concentration by counting back from ten to one, one number on each outbreath. Imagine each number as vividly as you can. Perhaps you can practically feel the number in your body. Ten, then nine...all the way back to one....

Every outbreath is an opportunity to relax and let go, to move into your Higher Self....Each outbreath is an opportunity to let go to a deeper and deeper state of wisdom, peace, and love....Now, listen to these new "what ifs" with the ears of your heart....Listen with every single cell of your body....

What if you weren't alone after all? What if you were a fragment of a great and glorious mind, like an individual wave is part of the magnificent ocean. Like an individual cell is part of the body. In your body, each cell has its own unique gift, its own special function that adds to the whole—and yet it also has the potential to become the whole. Any cell of your body could theoretically be cloned into a whole new you. Read this affirmation...

I am a child of the One Light, the One Mind.
The wisdom of the entire Universe is present within me.

What if your life is uniquely precious to the evolution of this universe? What if the Creator actually grows itself and knows itself through you, because you are love made visible. The life force is present in the dewy grass and the stars of the night sky. It is present in your mind and expresses through your creativity. You are the great and glorious dance of the One Great Dancer. You are the great and glorious dream of the One Great Dreamer. Listen to these affirmations, and if you wish, repeat them yourself.

God is present in all things, all experiences.
God is present within me.
The Universe knows itself and grows itself through me.

What if you didn't have to search for meaning in your life? What if you knew, with every fiber of your being, that the purpose of your life is to love? Through love you would find peace. And through peace you would see God in yourself, in your loved ones, in strangers, and in nature. If you believe that your purpose is to love, then you will stop judging yourself and others. This is forgiveness, and through forgiveness you will be free. Let these affirmations take root in your heart, repeating them if you wish.

The purpose of my life is to love.
I love by letting go of judgments.
Through forgiveness I find peace of mind.

What if the situations in your life that seem to bring up the most fear, frustration, and grief come in love's service? What if they are opportunities to wake up from the trance of your fears and your belief in separation? How could we find the light if not by struggling with the darkness? How could we become wise without making mistakes? How could we become compassionate toward others without suffering ourselves? Let these affirmations float in your mnd.

Darkness and fear are the Great Awakeners.
In facing my demons, I will find my freedom.

What if all your fears about death were based on a lie—the lie that you are a body? What if you had a body, but were not a body? Imagine that the coat of flesh you are sitting in is a spacesuit you have put on for an adventure in a strange, new world. Once you have returned from this adventure at the time of death, it will all rerun so that you can answer the question: Did I overcome fear and learn how to love? You don't have to wait until you take off your spacesuit to review your life. You can choose to wake up now. Listen to these affirmations, and repeat them if you wish.

I can wake up now.
I can choose to overcome fear by believing in love.

What if all the paradoxes and difficulties of life turn out to make sense after all? When we leave the confines of our spacesuits and return to a state where we can see forever, we will understand that every drama needed for the growth of our soul was provided for us. The circumstances of our lives reflected neither reward nor punishment, for we are neither good nor bad— we are just love growing itself. Listen to these affirmations, repeating them if you wish.

I am given the circumstances I require for my awakening.
Every situation, seen rightly, contains the seeds of
my freedom.

We like to think of the reframes you've just practiced as a kind of chiropractic adjustment of the attitude. As with all adjustments, this one is likely to slip over time. Our habitual ways of thinking are strong and tend to pull us back into old grooves through the force of habit. Eastern philosophies say that mind-habits called *samskaras* comprise the soul memories that we take with us at death. They are compared to riverbeds, carved through rock by the forceful stream of repetitive thinking. Overcoming the habitual samskara of fear is, as we have said before, a matter of developing a strong intention of practicing thought awareness so that you can make more creative choices.

One of the keys to reprogramming the mind with new choices is breathing. As I discuss at length in *Minding the Body, Mending the Mind*, breathing is the bridge between the body and the conscious mind. When breathing is slow and rhythmic, coming from the diaphragm, thoughts have true power because they are more deeply received as suggestion—not only by the mind, but also by the body. Yogis, Qi Gong masters, and martial arts experts all know how to use the breathing to stabilize the mind and energize the body.

Please stop for a moment and try this exercise before reading on. As you did before, either tape this exercise and play it back for yourself, or have someone read the script slowly and gently, pausing at the dots so that you have time to feel the words in your body.

DIAPHRAGMATIC (BELLY) BREATHING: The Foundation for Shifting from Fear to Love

Recline back in your chair at about a 45-degree angle. Now put one hand on your belly, and without trying to change your breathing in any way, notice whether your belly inflates as you breathe in and flattens as you breathe out, or whether some other movement predominates....For now, it doesn't matter how you are breathing. All that matters is your attention to the process.

Think of how babies breathe....Their bellies inflate like little beachballs on the inbreath and flatten on the out-

breath. They are breathing diaphrag-
matically—efficiently and restfully.
How about you? It may seem like your
belly is hardly moving at all....Or it may
seem like your belly is moving in the
opposite direction....Here's how to
make an easy shift into diaphragmatic
or belly breathing.

Take a big breath in, and now exhale
slowly and completely through your
mouth...that's right, really push it
out....Now, let the next breath come in
passively through your nose....Can you
feel your belly expand? Now, breathe
naturally through your nose, either
feeling or imagining the way that your
belly expands on the inbreath and
relaxes on the outbreath....This will
become second nature with a little
practice.

Throughout the day, you can learn to
take that big sigh of relief—the big outbreath...try it again right now...and
then notice the way that your breathing
moves into your belly. You can let go of
minor anxieties and bring forth the creative power of your mind by just concentrating on your breathing for a
minute or two, whatever else you may
be doing.

Do you feel more relaxed? While most people do, sometimes if you try too hard you can end up feeling a little tense for the first two or three times you practice the diaphragmatic breathing. But as soon as you catch on to it, you will have learned the single most important mental technique for interrupting fearful mental movies and coming back into the present moment.

Most of the fear in our life is not the result of old trauma or past-life soul impressions, although, as we will discuss in Chapter 18, transforming old wounds into wisdom is a crucial part of the healing process. Most of our fears are of the garden-variety type, created by the ways in which we think about common situations. Have you ever had the experience of dreading having to do something and then when the time came to do it, finding out that it was not so bad after all? In my own experience, I used to resist doing our income taxes for months. I wasted enormous mental energy in thinking about what a big chore the tax preparation would be. But when the day finally came, I could usually accomplish the entire dreaded task in a mere five or six hours. Too bad that I'd spent a few hundred hours ruminating about it!

Many of us can mobilize great fear and resistance to common problems such as traffic jams. There you are, safe in the car, but the dirty tricks department of the mind is producing movies about being late or right. Since none of these imaginings are going to move you one step closer to your destination, you might as well let go and come into the present moment. This is the time to take a big letting-go breath and shift into diaphragmatic or belly breathing. *Breathing is the gear-shift between fear and creativity.*

THREE KEYS TO CHANGING YOUR MIND

1. *Intention.* Think about a specific incident in which your fearful, judgmental thinking limited your ability to be creative and loving. This strengthens your intention to change. (Perhaps you yelled at one of your children, something you've done before, and you feel bad about it.)

2. *Awareness.* Notice when you are stuck in similar negative thoughts and judgments without putting yourself down. "Ah, I'm feeling critical. This is an opportunity to change my mind and open my heart."

3. *Creative Choice.* Shift into belly breathing. You are now in the present moment. What would a more creative choice be? "I can practice encouraging my daughter instead of criticizing her."

CHAPTER FOURTEEN

THE MEDITATIVE MIND

Before I sat down to write this chapter, I wandered through our gardens. The columbine were just coming into bloom, their blue and white faces a perfect complement to the border of pansies. Two spotted hawks rode the air currents, and a chorus of mountain bluebirds and jays greeted the morning. I felt like one of the Ute Indians who once held their summer festivals on the land where we live, savoring the summer fragrance of juniper and sage.

Although it was already hot by 8:00 A.M., a cool breeze wafted down from the snow fields that still cover the Continental Divide in late June. All around the house, wildflowers were in bloom. The deep blue of wild delphinium complemented the delicate pink of the profuse mountain geraniums. Yellow sedum seemed to peek out of every crevice in the rocky ledges that lead from the back of our house into the wilderness of Simpson's Gulch, where mountain lions, bears, and owls make their home.

Here in the front range of the Rocky Mountains, the landscape is subtle but ever-changing. If I'm *mindful*, present in the moment, it reveals itself ever more deeply. The colors seem to come alive, and the play of light and shadows reveal a world beyond the solid realm in which we live. At these moments—holy moments—I'm aware of drawing energy from both the earth and sky. I can sense the way that my life energy interpenetrates the rocks and trees and soars with the hawks and ravens. As I ride the tides of my breath, I am also aware that I am returning energy to the earth.

Stop for a moment and try this exercise. You can do it anywhere, but this time try it near a window, or better still, move outside. Either read through the directions until you feel comfortable trying the exercise, tape it for yourself, or have someone read the instructions to you.

AWARENESS TRAINING:
The Breath of Bridging Earth and Heaven

Sit with your feet flat on the ground and your back straight, yet relaxed.... Take a minute to stretch so that you feel as comfortable as possible in your body....Now allow your eyes to close.

Take a big letting-go breath, and then switch into belly breathing, feeling or imagining your belly expanding as you breathe in, and relaxing as you breathe out....Continue until you feel relaxed and present in your body....This is one of many ways to breathe. Now we will learn another way called the breath of bridging earth and heaven. We will imagine breathing energy from the sky and the earth simultaneously into the heart.

Let's start with breathing in the sky energy. Feel or imagine the energy of the sun above you—it doesn't matter whether it happens to be day or night as you do this....As you inhale, draw this energy in through the top of your head and into your heart. Breathe out a sense of spaciousness as if your breath could move out to the edges of the universe....Try this for several breaths....

Now we will breathe in the energy of the earth. Feel or imagine the earth energy beneath your feet....As you inhale, draw this energy in through your feet and up into your heart. Breathe out a sense of spaciousness as if your breath could move out to the edges of the universe....

Now we'll try the full breath of bridging earth and heaven. As you inhale, draw the sky energy down at the same time that you draw the earth energy up....Let them meet and mingle in your heart. Breathe out a sense of spacious awareness into the universe. Try this for a minute or two until you begin to get comfortable with it....

Now open your eyes and look out at nature. See the earth and the sky as you continue to do the breathing exercise. This breath brings you into the present moment and blesses the universe with your peaceful presence.

I use the breath of earth and heaven frequently to shift gears out of worried mind into mindfulness—a spacious awareness of the moment. At the end of the last chapter, we practiced the art of learning how to change our minds through *intention, awareness,* and *choice*. Breathing exercises—either belly breathing or the breath of earth and heaven—are the keys to this process. They represent the mental gearshift through which you move out of spinning your wheels into engaging the full power of your mind.

If your mental movies are mild, such as the irritation that can arise in a traffic jam, belly breathing is usually helpful in restoring sanity and allowing you to shift to a more creative mindset. But when mental movies are stronger, for example, if someone in the family is ill, belly breathing may not be enough to help you disengage your mental gears. In the latter circumstance, the breath of earth and heaven provides a stronger focus to help let go of persistent worries and return you to a more spacious outlook on life.

At a meditation retreat that Miron and I attended, the Tibetan Buddhist teacher Sogyal Rinpoche opened his arms wide. He smiled radiantly and said, "Meditation is being spacious." His arms opened wider still. "Meditation is being spacious and bringing the mind home." Perhaps you experienced a little bit of what Sogyal Rinpoche means in some of the exercises we have done together. When we are present in the moment, feeling our energy interpenetrate with earth and sky, we are comfortable in body and mind. We are at home in life. We feel part of something bigger, something infinitely comfortable and spacious. But when we begin to worry, our mind closes down like a fish grabbing a baited hook.

One winter, Miron and I were driving down a highway in New York State on our way to give a weekend retreat at the Phoenicia Pathwork Center. The sky was blue, and a wonderful blanket of snow covered the trees. I was feeling spacious and at home. Suddenly I thought about how infrequently we had skied that winter. The thought, "Other people who live in Colorado actually get to ski. Here we are working again," led to an avalanche of associated "poor me" thoughts. I was hooked. The infinite stream of the spacious present quickly faded as I began to suffer. Fortunately, in this instance, I was able to remember that I had a choice. I could return to enjoying the moment, or I could continue to suffer. A few minutes of the breath of bridging earth and heaven returned me to the spaciousness of the meditative mind. I was able to bring my mind home to the present.

The spacious mind is powerful because it reflects the Wholeness of our Higher Self. The constricted, worried mind is far less powerful. We all access the meditative state daily without making a particular effort. Whenever we feel comfortably absorbed in what we are doing, we are in the meditative mind. I usually feel that way when writing or gardening. In both cases, creative ideas flow freely, and I am often astounded by what comes through me. Miron feels particularly meditative and creative when he is at his art board drawing mandalas and other sacred pieces. Cooking and cleaning are very meditative for me, too, as long as there is no time pressure involved.

The Buddhist poet and writer, Thich Nhat Hanh, teaches his students to maintain a spacious, present awareness in whatever they are doing. Whether washing the dishes, driving a car, eating, or making love, mindfulness brings you fully to life. In his excellent book, *The Miracle of Mindfulness*, Thich Nhat Hanh suggests that you try bringing your full attention to different activities such as eating a tangerine, washing the dishes, or going for a walk. When you are finished with this period of reading, perhaps you might enjoy choosing one activity and doing it mindfully—with full attention.

I originally took up meditation for its medical benefits, discovering the deeper psychological and spiritual benefits much later. My nervous system was like a car that idled too high, always ready to respond to a threat. Since practically every interaction with another human being seemed threatening, I was in chronic overreaction to life. The simple diaphragmatic breathing exercise that you tried in the last chapter was the first type of meditation that I learned. I expanded this to a sitting meditation practice that consisted of counting back from four to one, for 10 or 20 minutes once or twice a day. This type of meditation, in which you are concentrating the mind on any repetitive stimulus, is called *concentration meditation*.

The physiological benefits of concentration meditation were first studied scientifically by doctors Herbert Benson and R. Keith Wallace. They found that Transcendental Meditation, which involves focusing on a mantra—or sacred sound—decreased heart rate, breathing rate, and oxygen consumption. These changes were accompanied by alterations in hormone levels and an increase in alpha waves in the cerebral cortex. They described these restful, restorative changes as a "wakeful hypometabolic state," which Benson subsequently termed *the relaxation response*—the physiological antidote to the fight-or-flight response. Benson went on to show that any simple kind of concentration meditation, whether secular or nonsecular, produced the same core of deeply restorative changes.

More recent research shows that under some conditions, deficient immune functions such as natural killer cell activity and helper T-cell function can be at least partially restored by simple concentration meditation. Benson's classic book, *The Relaxation Response*, documents the impressive effect of meditation on the cardiovascular system. The National Heart, Lung and Blood Institute of the National Institutes of Health now recommends meditation, exercise, stress management, and salt restriction as the first line of treatment for mild to moderate hypertension. Similarly, many irregularities of heart rhythm also respond to meditation. Amazingly, these beneficial changes occur after only a few weeks of practice, even in novice meditators who are almost always convinced that they are doing the meditation incorrectly!

For example, when we ask people at workshops to raise their hands if they meditate, a lot of people usually respond. But when we ask them to keep their hands up if they think they are meditating "well," most of the hands go down. The mind is actually a very busy place, jumping from thought to thought like a wild monkey. Typically, you will lose your focus and get lost in thought, only to "come to" a minute or two later and think, "Uh-oh, I was supposed to be meditating." *This is absolutely natural.*

Sogyal Rinpoche compares the mind to an ocean. Just as it is the nature of the ocean to rise and fall in waves, it is the nature of the mind to rise and fall in thoughts. Thoughts are always arising and then passing away again. Even skillful meditators still think. The difference between them and novice meditators is that skillful meditators no longer get upset about thinking.

The skillful meditator begins to think about her job and simply notices, "Thinking, thinking." She lets go and returns to the meditation. The ocean of her mind is making waves, and knowing that this is completely natural, she lets them be. The novice meditator, in contrast, begins to think and may then say, "Oh, my mind is so active. I'm always thinking. I'm not supposed to be thinking. This is awful...." Dr. Benson counsels his patients to take an "Oh, well" attitude towards thinking. It doesn't matter. It's just the mind making waves.

Let me give you an example of a typical meditation. Let's say you have chosen to focus on breathing and counting back repetitively from four to one. Perhaps you get down to one and notice that you are feeling a little more relaxed. Then the inner dialogue may begin, "Boy, this meditation is great. Just four breaths and I'm relaxed already....Why is it that something so easy is so hard to make time for...." Thinking, thinking..."four, three, two, one, four, three, two, one, four..."my waistband seems a little bit tight. I bet I'm gaining weight again. I watch what I eat, but I don't have time to exercise—and that knee never recovered from skiing last year. Not that we'll go much this year, it's so expensive"....And then you catch yourself again. Thinking, thinking. "Four, three, two, one..." this is how it goes.

Meditation is a type of mental martial arts training in which we learn to side-step the ego and its incessant judging. Every time you let go and return to your concentration, the mental muscles of awareness and choice are being exercised. Remarkably, even when most of a meditation exercise is spent thinking, beneficial bodily changes still occur. I think of that as a sort of grace. Even the intention to let go produces a near-magical result. When meditation is discontinued, the physical benefits generally disappear within a few weeks. But why make meditation an all-or-nothing thing? Some people enjoy sitting for 10 or 20 or 30 minutes with closed eyes, and some don't. You can just as easily take several mini meditation breaks throughout the day, shifting to belly breathing, the breath of bridging earth and heaven, or the lovingkindness meditation we will learn in Chapter 15.

When I still worked at the Mind/Body Clinic, we used to send follow-up questionnaires to our patients six months after they had completed the ten-week program. While the majority no longer sat for regular 10- to 20-minute periods of meditation, almost all of them practiced mindfulness as part of daily life, and a majority of those still experienced relief from the physical symptoms that had first brought them to the clinic. Meditation is not just a practice, it is a way of life. Initially, that way of life is learned through formal practice, just as we learn to play a musical instrument in this fashion. Some people will choose to continue practice periods and others won't, but both will have shifted the paradigm through which they relate to the world.

Unless you have had a formal meditation practice at another time, we recommend that you start one now and continue for a minimum of three months with regular daily discipline. You might choose concentration meditation, mindfulness of breathing, a body form of meditation such as hatha yoga or tai chi, repetitive prayer, walking meditation, or any practice that you feel drawn to. The easiest way to establish a routine for meditation is to choose the same time each day. Many people simply get up 20 minutes earlier in the morning and meditate before the momentum of the day carries them away. If you simply "look for" 20 minutes here and there, you will rarely find them, just as you won't save much money if your strategy is to put aside whatever is left at the end of the week. Your intention to establish a regular routine is the most important asset you can bring to your practice.

Our good friend Robin Casarjian, author of *Forgiveness:A Bold Choice for a Peaceful Heart*, teaches prisoners how to meditate. She tells them the amazing story of a prisoner in a Chinese concentration camp who attributed his sanity and health after 10 years in solitary confinement to his daily meditation practice. The most fascinating part of this story was the man's statement that he really had to make a strong effort to find the time to meditate each day! So, if it's hard to put aside the time when you're in solitary confinement, no wonder we have to make such an effort to do it in the busy-ness of the outside world, even if our physical lives depend upon it.

Mindfulness meditation was first introduced as a medical treatment by Dr. Jon Kabat-Zinn, who founded the Stress Reduction and Relaxation Clinic at the University of Massachusetts Medical School in Worcester in the late 1970s. The remarkable results of his 10-week program are detailed in his excellent book, *Full Catastrophe Living*. Jon calls mindfulness "being fully awake in our lives." Dr. Kabat-Zinn was very helpful to us when we were setting up our Mind/Body Clinic at the Beth Israel Hospital. It was from his program, which was an early model for our own, that we learned the tremendous power of mindfulness meditation in working with both physical and emotional pain.

Dr. Kabat-Zinn's clinic was featured on the popular Bill Moyers series, *Healing and the Mind*, which aired on PBS television stations in 1993. In one very touching sequence, he was coaching a woman on how to practice a hatha yoga posture mindfully. She was in so much pain that a tear escaped her eye. Rather than telling her to get up and rest, Jon helped her become present to the pain, to go into it rather than avoiding it, while wiping away her tears.

Our mind generally tries to escape from both physical and emotional pain, but if the pain is persistent, it keeps gnawing away at the edges of consciousness. As a result, muscles tense to keep the pain at bay, and both mental and physical energy is depleted. In contrast, when you choose to become mindfully aware of the pain, resistance diminishes. Instead of feeling like the victim of the pain, you become its observer, and there is a world of difference between those two positions!

In workshops, we often demonstrate the powerful way that mindfulness can change the experience of pain. Participants close their eyes and scan their bodies until they find an area of pain or tension. Adopting the stance of a curious detective, they pay close attention to every sensation that arises and then passes away without judging or commenting on the sensations. As soon as we label a sensation "pain," or think "it's killing me," the body/mind responds to our thought.

Pain is actually made up of two components: the *physical sensation* and *our thoughts about the sensation*. Even if the former stays the same, our perception of the pain can change dramatically by altering the latter. The spacious awareness of mindfulness brings the mind home and frees it from the hook of painful thoughts.

Stop and try this exercise before reading on. *As usual, you may want to read it through and then try it from memory, tape it for yourself, or have another person read the exercise slowly, pausing at the dots to let you enter the experience fully.*

MINDFULNESS OF TENSION

Take a moment to stretch so that you feel as fully present in your body as possible....Now, allow your eyes to close and take a big letting-go breath....Shift your breathing either to the belly or to the breath of bridging earth and heaven....

Now, allow yourself to become aware of your body. There are probably some very comfortable areas, while other places may feel tense or painful....
Choose a tense or painful area, and imagine that you can breathe directly into that spot....Let the breath come and go from that place while you notice everything you can about the sensations there.... Be like a detective, noticing every nuance of feeling, of energy flow....You can do this without mental commentary or judgment.

Try letting the sensations just be rather than labeling them as good or bad....Just be present to what is....Continue this exercise for a minute or two until you feel ready to come back and open your eyes.

What did you experience? It's common to notice that tension or pain intensifies when we bring our awareness to it. But then the sensation often changes and either diminishes or even disappears. On the very rare occasions when I get a migraine headache, I rest and use the pain as a focus for mindfulness meditation. It is so interesting! First, there may be a shooting sensation, followed by a wave of nausea. For a while everything seems calm, and then I might feel throbbing in one temple that quickly shifts to an ache in the jaw. Next I may feel pressure in the eye, which gives way to a warm sense of pleasure and then settles into a toothache. And after a while, the pain may stop or I may fall asleep.

Before I learned to meditate, my response to a migraine was very different. First, I'd get angry. Why did this have to happen to me? Then I'd feel envious of all the people who were going about their business while I lay in a dark room vomiting and writhing in pain. Oftentimes, I'd cry both from the intensity of the pain and from plain old self-pity. The harder I cried, the worse the pain became. As a child, the pain was so intense that on several occasions I even contemplated suicide. I definitely felt victimized. Now my perception is completely different. A migraine is an opportunity to rest and meditate. It's not pleasant, but it's not that unpleasant either. It's just what's happening. I can be spacious about it.

So, what is meditation? Essentially, it's about being spacious and bringing the mind home.

CHAPTER FIFTEEN

PRACTICAL TIPS ON MEDITATION

I was trying to meditate in an easy chair by our living room window early one morning in the mid-1970s. The kids kept running by, sometimes stopping to engage me in conversation. Then the phone rang. I didn't get up to answer it, but on every successive ring, I worried that it could be my parents. It was early to call unless some disaster had occurred. By the time Miron had picked up the phone, my mind was already engaged in disaster fantasies. They continued after he'd hung up. Not only was my undisciplined mind noisy, even the refrigerator seemed more raucous than usual that morning. I was having real trouble "bringing my mind home." When two-year-old Andrei bit Justin in the ankle and they both began to scream, I got up in terminal disgust. Our home and my mind both felt like Grand Central Station.

Far from feeling spacious, I was frustrated and angry. As I made my way into the kitchen, mumbling under my breath, a lovely woman named Daya, who lived with us at that time, came out for breakfast. When I told her how upset I was, she gave me a wise smile. "You don't find many yogis meditating on the subway, even though they could. Even people who have learned to master their minds still take care of themselves by finding a quiet place for prayer and meditation." Her words hit home. I was approaching meditation the way I did the rest of my life. I was trying to meditate *and* be there for the kids, once again forgetting that I had to take time for myself.

From that day on, I meditated in a quieter place. Since our house was small, a corner of the bedroom was the only space I could liberate, and even then, I had to negotiate with Miron and the children for "alone" time there. When your family is used to having you accessible all the time, they may not respect your need for complete peace and quiet. I approached this challenge by teaching the kids to meditate through belly breathing and progressive muscle relaxation. Although their attention span was limited, they enjoyed themselves if we kept the exercise short. Then when it was time for me to meditate alone, they were my allies. They knew what I was doing. The rule about meditators in our house is simple: Don't disturb except in case of fire or blood.

I was fortunate in having Daya and other meditation teachers around to ask for advice. Certain questions like where and when to meditate, what to do about falling asleep, and how to manage one's thoughts come up for almost everyone. We'd like to take the opportunity to address some of these questions now.

When Is the Best Time to Practice?

As we discussed in the last chapter, meditation is a discipline in the same way that saving money is. You need to put aside some attention for it each day on a *regular schedule*. Many people find that meditating the first thing in the morning, before the day gets going, works well. Other people enjoy meditating before dinner, and some before bed. The key is to find a time when you are alert and most likely to be undisturbed. Since blood flow is diverted from the brain to the gut after eating, wait about two hours after a big meal to meditate; otherwise you are likely to fall asleep.

While I'm usually too sleepy before bed to meditate regularly at this time, I always go to sleep meditating. It sure beats ruminating over my anxieties! If you decide not to continue a regular practice after committing to a three-month training period, meditating your way to sleep will continue to keep the practice alive for you. In addition, if you wake up during the night, meditation can help put you back to sleep. And even if you don't fall back to sleep, you will have benefited from a period of deep rest.

What Is the Correct Posture?

It's easiest to meditate if your spine is straight and your body posture is symmetrical. If you are meditating while falling asleep, naturally you will be lying down. But since lying down favors sleep, it is not recommended for meditation at other times. Pay attention to your posture now as I describe how to sit. You can sit in a chair with both feet on the floor. Most people find that if they get too comfortable in a plush chair, they nod off. So, choose a simple chair with a straight back. Put both feet on the ground, and either put one hand on each knee or rest your hands in your lap. You may also want to sit on the floor cross-legged. In that case, put a firm cushion—not a bed pillow—under your backside to support your spine. Otherwise you will have to fight the tendency to fall backwards. Experiment with different cushions until you find one that supports you effortlessly and comfortably.

If I Exercise, Is It Best to Meditate Before or After?

If you generally exercise, try doing it before meditation. Since you've just expended energy, your body/mind will naturally move into a recovery cycle quite conducive to the meditative state. Whether or not you've just exercised, it is always a good idea to relax and let go of any tension that is stored in your muscles before you begin meditating. Tense muscles make for a racing mind. Soft muscles make for a spacious mind. If you feel particularly tense, try a hot shower or bath first.

I Fall Asleep Whenever I Try to Meditate. What's Wrong?

Miron and I have a cartoon that shows two monks meditating. One is sitting up straight, and the other is falling over. The caption reads, "There is a fine line between meditating and napping." While studies indicate that even advanced meditators sleep for about 20 percent of their practice time, when the scale tips to 50 percent or more, you've been napping, not meditating. In the first few weeks of meditation, it is very common to nod off. After all, you're used to falling asleep when you relax your muscles and disengage your mind. It takes time to train yourself to maintain a state of consciousness that is both relaxed and alert.

As long as the room is not too warm and your posture is erect, you'll soon be able to stay awake unless you're so exhausted that your body will take any opportunity for a catnap. Sometimes we're so tired and push ourselves so hard, that when we finally take time out, we just fall asleep. In this case, listen to the advice of your body and get more sleep at other times so that you will be alert for meditation.

Avoidance of emotional pain is the other common reason for falling asleep. Many new meditators don't like sitting down with nothing to do and no place to go because their anxieties seem to intensify. Normally, we are moving targets for our own fear. If it gets oppressive, we can always phone a friend, read a book, watch TV, have a snack, take a walk, or otherwise distract ourselves. Not so when we meditate. Part of learning the mental martial arts required to transform fear is to sit still and be aware of it. This may initially feel strange and uncomfortable if we have spent much of our life running from anxieties.

Meditation Exhausts Me. Am I Trying Too Hard?

Meditation is often called an "effortless effort." What a paradox! Do you remember what a Chinese finger trap is? You stick a finger in each end of a woven, straw tube and then try to pull each finger out. The harder you try, the more stuck you get. The same principle applies to meditation. To succeed, you need to relax and let go. Primarily, this means not judging yourself and not trying too hard. Meditation is a state of being, not an act of doing. When your mind wanders, just notice impassively. Don't start judging yourself as a no-good meditator.

One woman who had completed our ten-week Mind/Body course came back six months later for an eight-week "graduate group." Sometime during those six months, her meditation practice had made the shift into effortless effort. She explained to the group, "I finally realized that meditation wasn't about doing anything. I just sit there." This was very freeing for the rest of the group. Remember that the only definition of a "good" meditation is one that you sat down and did.

My Mind Wanders So Much That I Wonder If I'm Getting Anything Out of Meditation.

I often compare the wandering mind to toddlers who are running off from their mother's side to smell the flowers. While Mother is delighted by the curiosity of her children, she also knows that they need to keep walking. So, with great respect and love, she brings them back to the path and they continue. The children are not "wrong" for wandering off; it is their nature. The wandering mind is really a great opportunity because you repeatedly practice bringing it back to focus, strengthening the mental muscles of awareness and letting go.

Many people suffer from the illusion that every other meditator is in bliss, and they are the only ones thinking about what to eat for dinner. As we discussed in the last chapter, the wandering mind is absolutely natural. The challenge is to be like the good mother who gently brings her toddlers back. Studies of novice meditators indicate that physiological benefits still occur even when the meditators thinks that their minds have just been wandering. As long as you continue to practice for 10 to 20 minutes a day, at least 3 times a week, most likely you are bringing forth the relaxation response in spite of your busy mind.

There Are So Many Different Types of Meditation. How Do I Know Which One Is Right for Me?

There are as many ways to meditate as there are human beings. When people tell me that they have tried to meditate but can't get into it, I know that they just haven't found a practice that suits them. One person may be drawn to a sitting practice of mindfulness, another to repetitive prayer such as the rosary. One person may find that awareness of the body and breath while swimming or running is his or her preferred form of meditation, another may be drawn to yoga, tai chi, or mindful walking. In all instances, the "formal" meditation is only a training for approaching every moment of life like a meditation.

Look over the list of meditations that follows. These are meant to supplement the basic practices of breath-centered concentration, meditation, and mindfulness through the breath of bridging earth and heaven that we have learned previously. If any of them seem appealing to you, give them a try. It is preferable to work with a meditation for several days before you decide that it is not for you. There is always a period of adjustment to anything new, and if we give up before the adjustment is over, we may have lost a great opportunity.

1. Centering Prayer

Centering prayer is a form of meditation that represents a conscious decision to let go of the limitations of the ego and open up to the unlimited mind of God. This form of meditation has been popularized by Father Thomas Keating, a Cistercian monk and the abbot of the Snowmass Monastery in Colorado. In centering prayer, we shift awareness away from the thoughts that Keating compares to boats floating down the river of consciousness to the river itself. The river is the Divine Presence. Keating's book, *Open Heart, Open Mind,* is an excellent primer on the art of centering prayer. While centering prayer is not a breath-focused form of meditation, I have preceded the standard instructions for centering prayer with a few minutes of breath-awareness to ease you into the inner silence:

> *Focus* your mind by counting back from four to one on successive out-breaths....Continue for two or three minutes....
>
> *Now* let go of counting, and let your awareness focus on the feelings of peace and tranquility that naturally arise as your mind begins to quiet down.
>
> *When* you begin to think, mentally repeat a word or phrase of your choice—what Keating calls a prayer word. Examples of prayer words might

be *thank you, peace, shalom, Kyrie Eleison, om, love*—whatever word inspires you to an awareness of the Divine Presence. Keating makes the point that the word itself is unimportant. Its power comes from reminding you of your intention to let go of ego and become fully aware of God.

As soon as your mind quiets down, let go of the prayer word and sit quietly in the inner silence. Continue for as long as you like.

2. Holy Moment Meditation

I often start my meditations by recalling a holy moment because it brings forth the very feelings of spacious awareness that are the hallmarks of meditation. You can also use this recollection as a meditation in its own right.

Take a few letting-go breaths, and remember a time when you felt present in the moment—absorbed in a sunset, marveling at fresh-fallen snow, enchanted by the smile of a baby....If several memories come, choose just one....

Enter the memory with all of your senses. Remember the sights and colors...the fragrances...the position and movement of your body...the emotional or felt sense....

Let the memory go and meditate on the feelings that remain—the stillness and joy of your own Higher Self....

3. Lovingkindness (Metta) Meditation

This is one of my favorite forms of meditation. You can do it as your entire practice or at the end of a period of meditation. You can also do little mini-lovingkindness meditations during the day, sending blessings to people.

Begin by taking a few letting-go breaths and start to quiet down by focusing on either belly breathing or the breath of bridging earth and heaven.

Imagine a Great Star of Light above you and slightly in front of you, pouring a waterfall of love and light over you. Let the light enter the top of your head and wash through you, revealing the purity of your own heart, which expands and extends beyond you, merging with the Divine Light. See yourself totally enclosed in the Egg of Light and then repeat these lovingkindness blessings for yourself, with all the respect and love that you would have for your only child:

May I be at peace,
May my heart remain open,
May I awaken to the light of my
own true nature, May I be healed,
May I be a source of healing
for all beings.

~

Next, bring one or more loved ones to mind. See them in as much detail as possible, imagining the loving Light shining down on them and washing through them, revealing the light within their own hearts. Imagine this light growing brighter, merging with the Divine Light, and enclosing them in the Egg of Light. Then bless them:

May you be at peace,
May your heart remain open,
May you awaken to the light of
your own true nature,
May you be healed,
May you be a source of
healing for all beings.

Repeat these blessings for as many people as you wish.

~

Next, think of a person or persons whom you hold in judgment, and to whom you're ready to begin extending forgiveness. Place them in the Egg of Light, and see the Light washing away all their negativity and illusions, just as it did for you and your loved ones. Bless them:

May you be at peace,
May your heart remain open,
May you awaken to the light of
your own true nature,
May you be healed,
May you be a source of
healing for all beings.

See our beautiful planet as it appears from outer space, a delicate jewel spinning in the starry vastness of space. Imagine the earth surrounded by light—the green continents, the blue waters, the white polar caps, the two-leggeds and four-leggeds, the fish that swim, and the birds that fly. Earth is a realm of opposites. Of day and night, good and evil, sickness and health, riches and poverty, up and down, male and female. Be spacious enough to hold it all as you offer these blessings:

May there be peace on earth,
May the hearts of all people be open to
themselves and to each other,
May all people awaken to the light
of their own true nature,
May all creation be blessed and
be a blessing to All That Is.

≈

4. Walking Meditation

Sometimes your mind may be too busy for a sitting meditation, particularly if you are in the midst of adjusting to an illness or other challenge. For many years, I found that hatha yoga was the best form of meditation for me because the sensations of breathing and stretching gave me a firm anchor for my troubled mind. Some people enjoy tai chi or other forms of moving meditation instead of, or in addition to, sitting forms. One of the most universally delightful practices is walking meditation. The Vietnamese Buddhist monk, Thich Nhat Hanh, has popularized this wonderful activity.

Find someplace in nature to walk.

Begin by focusing on your breathing and the sensation of walking. Notice the movements of your feet—how each one lifts, moves forward in space, and then descends again.

Let your awareness expand beyond the physical sensation of walking to the beauty all around you. Keep about 25 percent of your awareness on breathing, and about 75 percent on a spacious awareness of everything you see, hear, feel, and smell.

Just as in a sitting meditation, when you begin thinking, let go and return to an awareness of breath and mindfulness.

CHAPTER SIXTEEN

CREATIVE IMAGINATION AND HYPNOSIS

People often wonder about the difference between meditation and hypnosis. Psychologist and writer Jeanne Achterberg often speaks about the case of a young girl who was kidnapped, raped, and tortured in the early 1980s. I remember reading about that terrible tragedy and hearing about it for weeks on the news. After raping the girl, the kidnapper cut off both her arms and left her for dead. Miraculously, she walked miles to safety without bleeding to death even though both radial arteries were severed. When asked how she managed to save herself, the girl replied that she thought of herself as the bionic woman, an invincible character in a popular television show of the time.

This young girl, who survived through the power of imagining herself bionic, had inadvertently used an indirect form of hypnosis to staunch the flow of blood. While meditation has to do with emptying our minds of images, bringing forth the nonspecific healing physiology of the relaxation response, hypnosis is about creating vivid mental images that our bodies respond to specifically.

About one in twenty people are so capable of absorbing themselves in fantasy that their bodies can respond like that of the girl mentioned above. All of us respond somewhat to mental pictures when we blush, get goosebumps, or experience sexual arousal through fantasy. And even a moderate ability to use our imaginations can help tremendously in the healing process.

Children hospitalized in burn units must endure the pain of debridement when dead skin is scrubbed off the surface of their wounds to hasten the process of healing. When skin grafting is necessary, sometimes the grafts take, but other times they are sloughed off. Both the pain of debridement and the chance of a graft taking can be positively affected by hypnosis. Some children can be helped to relax and then given the direct hypnotic suggestion that their burned area feels completely numb and comfortable. Through hypnosis they can achieve partial or even complete control of pain during and even after debridement. An indirect form of hypnosis can also help these children's skin grafts take. Children who are shown informational diagrams about graft attachment in which little hands from the graft bed reach up and connect with little hands coming down from the skin graft have a significantly better chance of successful grafts. Their minds automatically incorporate the idea that healing is in the process of occurring.

Psychologist Neil Fiore wrote a marvelous letter to the prestigious *New England Journal of Medicine* when he was recovering from treatment for testicular cancer. He noticed that when you become a patient, you automatically enter a highly hypnotizable state. All your senses are focused on getting information that has to do with staying alive. That's a powerful focus! When any information relevant to survival is presented, the mind pounces on it. Even casual comments by the receptionist, noted Fiore, can be effective hypnotic suggestions. He wanted the whole health care team to know how their slightest word, gesture, or facial expression sinks directly into the mind of the patient as an indirect hypnotic suggestion.

Under normal circumstances, our minds tend to be scattered. We think about so many different things that none of them has much power. In this state, images come and go like a light snow that immediately blows off the road. But when the mind focuses, images can become deeply imbedded in the body/mind like a heavy, sticking snow. A casual comment to a person who is sick can thus be a strong hypnotic suggestion. For example, when a person with a life-threatening illness is invited to go to a winter coat sale in August, the image that forms is one of surviving through winter! As we imagine ourselves reaching future goals, healing images are being sent indirectly to the body.

When Karmu the healer messed with Miron's mind by having him soak in a bathtub of purple medicine for 11 minutes, he was employing an indirect form of hypnosis to cure a cold. The novel situation focused Miron's mind and made it receptive to changing his paradigm, or usual hypnotic mindset, from helplessness and pessimism to optimism and limitless possibility. The resultant changes in neuropeptides, blood flow, immune measures, and other physiological processes resulted in an immediate cure of Miron's cold, even though the cold, per se, was never mentioned!

A more direct approach might have involved suggestions to mobilize Miron's white cells to destroy cold viruses. There is currently no research that speaks to the particular efficacy of either direct or indirect methods of hypnosis for healing from major illness. We have always felt that if a person feels particularly drawn to a certain type of healing image, then it's best to follow that intuitive lead. We're often asked whether an anatomically correct healing image is superior to a symbolic one. The best image is simply the one that feels most alive to you, whether it's a direct image of a microscopically detailed killer cell poking holes in a tumor cell, a knight spearing the enemy, or an image of attending your daughter's college graduation in seven more years.

One of the potential down-sides of using imagery for healing is the inadvertent creation of a life-or-death battle. When teaching imagery to cancer patients, I've noticed that some people get very excited and energized by the idea of their immune system conquering cancer cells. Other people find imagery a struggle. Either it doesn't seem appealing, or it actually becomes frightening because they keep wondering, "Am I doing this right? Am I helping myself enough? Will it be my own fault if I die? Could I be hurting myself by thinking wrong?" When Miron and I toured Australia with the recovered cancer patient, Dr. Ian Gawler, Ian gave a tremendous demonstration of how indirect negative imagery can subvert the entire healing process. He asked a group of workshop participants to close their eyes and meditate on anything they wanted other than a black horse. *Close your eyes and try that for a minute. Hard, isn't it? Now close your eyes and meditate on a red rose.*

The black horse represents not dying. When your efforts to heal are focused on the fear of death, when you are trying to keep death from happening, paradoxically you focus intently on it. So, when imagery techniques or any technique is done to prevent death, we indirectly create ongoing images of black horses. The red rose, on the other hand, represents a focus on life. When we use imagery or any other technique to live life with more creativity, joy, and love, we automatically enhance indirect healing imagery. It may be that a black horse will gallop through our rose field from time to time, but it isn't our major preoccupation. We are not hypnotized by it. We're not saying that Ian's strategy is right for everybody. Only you know whether you will feel empowered by the use of specific healing images or whether they might indirectly bring up images of death or failure.

Our son Andrei gave us a delightful lesson in the use of creative imagination and hypnosis when he was only six. We had just returned from a visit to the pediatrician, who had checked the bottom of Andrei's left foot and recommended surgery for a large, painful plantar wart. We felt frightened by the prospect of surgery and were motivated to try other things first. Miron and I knew the work of Harvard psychiatrist Owen Surman, who had conducted meticulous experiments on hypnosis and remission of warts. Warts, it seems, respond very well to suggestion. A delightful variety of ancient healing techniques including applying moss collected at the full moon are known to sometimes cure warts. Surman reasoned that the warts were really cured by the placebo effect, an indirect form of hypnosis brought about by belief in the efficacy of a treatment. He conducted an experiment with people who had intractable warts that previous treatments had not cured and sure enough, under hypnosis, over half the people were cured!

Bolstered by Surman's study data, Miron and I decided to hypnotize Andrei. The problem was that neither of us knew a thing about hypnosis. We had visions of hanging a crystal on a string and swinging it back and forth in front of him until he began to follow it like a cobra in a snakecharmer's basket. At that point, we reasoned, he would be in a trance, and we could offer some direct hypnotic suggestions for disappearance of the warts. Andrei, however, had no interest at all in playing the snake to my charmer. So, in a burst of inspiration, I told Andrei that we were going to teach him a magical wart-removal incantation. Kids like magic, so that got his attention.

Very solemnly, we had him pick up his foot and cradle it in his two hands. He was then told to close his eyes and repeat, "Begone, begone, begone wart. Begone in the name of Jesus Christ, Amen," three times. This wart exorcism was repeated religiously every night before bed. In a week the wart had begun to turn black as its blood supply dried up. A few weeks later, it fell off and left a bed of new, pink skin. Andrei was very pleased with himself and for several years thereafter we occasionally heard mumbling behind closed doors about "begone" this or that. He generalized his wart healing prayer to colds, chicken pox, and other assorted maladies!

Unfortunately, when Andrei reached adolescence, his childhood experience seemed somehow naive or silly to him, and he lost the power to heal through the magic of his mind. Perhaps Jesus had a story or two such as this one in mind when he commented that only when we become as little children shall we enter the Kingdom of Heaven. To children all things are possible. To the Creator all things are possible. For us to co-create the Universe, we must indeed become again as little children. Entering into the meditative mind, the space of limitless possibility, is one way to become as little children. The other way, as we will begin to explore in the next chapter, is to face our fears and transform the wounds that limit our perception into a universal sense of compassion and creativity.

At workshops, people often ask us the difference between hypnosis and meditation. At the most basic level, meditation is the removal of all mindsets so that we can perceive the world freshly, as it is. Hypnosis, in contrast, is the cultivation of a particular mindset. Guided imagery exercises may incorporate meditation as well as both direct and indirect forms of hypnosis. Dr. Herbert Benson studied the physiology of the induction phase of hypnosis. The induction phase of classical, direct hypnosis is generally a period of relaxation or focus on the breathing that disengages our mental gears from outer concerns and delivers us into a state of focused, open attention. In other words, the induction phase is similar to meditation and elicits the same physiological response, the so-called relaxation response.

In the relaxed, aware state of meditation, we are most open to the power of the imagination. The relaxation response is like a doorway into other mental/physiological states. Once we go through that doorway, our bodies can respond in remarkable ways to suggestion. If touched by a finger that we are told is a hot poker, our skin may redden or even blister. Some people can inhibit or augment their body's immune response to substances such as tuberculin. Yogis can stop their breathing and heart rate so they appear dead, yet can "come back to life" hours or even days later. These changes clearly go beyond the core changes of the relaxation response.

In the late 1970s, I came across a wonderful book that I purchased for a dime at a garage sale. It was entitled *Magic and Mystery in Tibet*, by Alexandra David-Neel. I sat riveted as I read David-Neel's account of dressing like a man and actually sneaking into a Tibetan monastery to study. She reported some remarkable feats of creative imagination that she had seen the monks perform. Tibet once had a tradition of long-distance running called Longompa. The runners, however, prepared in a way totally antithetical to sports physiology. They meditated for years, using complex visualizations, while sitting in the bottom of ten-foot-deep holes. They were ready for competition when they could levitate out of the ground! That practice certainly caught my imagination.

Another practice that David-Neel described was called gTumo yoga. In Tibetan, gTumo means "fierce woman" and refers to the Qi or kundalini energy. This fiery energy is visualized running through certain subtle channels to purify people's negativity and bring them to spiritual awakening. A by-product of this practice is the liberation of intense heat. David-Neel described how gTumo practitioners were draped in wet sheets during a festival that falls on the full moon each February. Sitting in the cold, at high elevations in the Himalayas, they were able to dry several sheets in the course of the evening's prayers due to the heat caused by gTumo visualizations.

I was a postdoctoral fellow in Behavioral Medicine at Harvard Medical School at the time that I was reading David-Neel's book. My mentor, Herbert Benson, who was interested in studying advanced forms of meditation, found gTumo fascinating. Shortly after we had discussed it, his holiness the Dalai Lama came to Harvard, and we had the good fortune to meet him. He and Dr. Benson had a lively conversation concerning the physiological benefits and possibilities of meditation. When asked whether there were any practitioners of Longompa left, he laughed with his characteristically twinkling style and remarked that Longompa is no longer needed. We have airplanes now!

There are, however, still practitioners of gTumo, and his holiness allowed Dr, Benson and several other scientists to come to Dharamsala in India to study them. Their experiments indicated that the Tibetan monks could indeed raise their body temperatures more than ten degrees externally, although their core—or inner—temperature remained unchanged. Similar changes can be accomplished through biofeedback by simply asking people to "think warm." One interesting experiment performed by the U.S. Army Corps of Engineers concerned gloves for Arctic climates. Men were put into a cold chamber under three conditions: thin leather gloves alone, thin leather gloves with the instruction "think warm," and Arctic gloves. The men in the thin leather gloves who were told to "think warm" had hand temperatures equivalent to those in Arctic gear. It is a relief that we don't have to be accomplished yogis to use the power of our minds in ways that can help our bodies.

Meditation is also often used as a clinical treatment for Reynaud's disease, a condition in which the capillaries of the extremities constrict, with the result that hands and feet are cold, painful, and sometimes even blue. Some of my patients actually had to wear gloves in the supermarket when walking down the frozen food aisle. When they learned how to "think warm," bringing to mind images of sitting in a hot bath or plunging their hands into warm sand, the gloves were no longer necessary. Similarly, hand-warming frequently cuts down on both the incidence and severity of migraine headaches. (There are several excellent books on the use of guided imagery for healing listed in the resources section.)

If you have any doubt about the power of imagination to affect your body, try this experiment.

Take a few letting-go breaths and allow your eyes to close. Now imagine that you are in the kitchen, opening your refrigerator. There on the top shelf is the biggest, juiciest yellow lemon you have ever seen. Take it out and feel its weight in your hand. What is the texture like? The color? Can you locate the end where the stem once was? Lift the lemon to your nose and smell it. Now scrape the lemon with a fingernail and smell it again. Is there a difference? Can you feel the lemon oil where the skin has been scraped? Now imagine taking the lemon over to a cutting board, picking up a sharp knife and cutting it neatly in half. Pick up one of the halves and watch the juice welling up. Now stick out your tongue and lick the lemon.

Did you notice any physiological response? Sometimes I pucker up in anticipation of doing that exercise, before I've actually imagined anything in particular. Our bodies respond not only to visual images but to simple thought. Some people can see in technicolor. Others see little or nothing, but they might have a particularly well-developed sense of touch or hearing, smell, or taste. Each one of us imagines in our own way. However your imagination works is fine. Can you remember the last time you ate at a restaurant? Whether you flashed on the taste, the emotions you felt, the sounds or the sights, doesn't matter. You had your own way of accessing the memory. This is all you require to use the power of the imagination for healing.

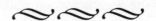

CHAPTER SEVENTEEN

WAKING FROM THE DREAM:
A Psychospiritual Framework for Healing

Have you ever seen a side-show demonstration in which a hypnotist chooses a strait-laced member of the audience, puts him in a trance, and then makes him cluck like a chicken? Perhaps the greatest fear people have about hypnosis is losing control of their minds to an outside force. As a nine-year-old, I angrily resisted the ministrations of a hypnotist hired by a friend's mother to entertain us at a birthday party. "You can't control me," I fumed. Sadly, we're all already controlled by hypnotic images implanted early in life by parents, friends, clergy, the media, teachers, and seemingly random events. We all have myths that guide us, life stories to which we are profoundly attached, and we continue to act in these stories like characters in a dream. The hypnotist who controls us is not outside us, but within.

Consider the strange and disturbing case of Amanda, a social worker who literally felt that she was living in a dream. She often lost hours or days from conscious awareness and had no idea where the time had gone. Sometimes she would wake up in a strange hotel room and not understand how she had gotten there or what she had been doing. After one episode, she arrived home to find her husband in a state of panic. No one knew where she had gone. Later in the month, when the credit card bills arrived, Amanda was shocked to find charges that she couldn't recall making. It turned out that Amanda's body had gone on a spending spree, bought a new wardrobe, and then enjoyed three days of gambling in Las Vegas—activities that the quiet, frugal Amanda had absolutely no interest in.

Under hypnosis with a skilled psychiatrist, a personality called Shelly emerged and took over Amanda's body. Shelly had a smile that could light up the room in contrast to Amanda's very shy, tentative demeanor. Leaning back seductively in her chair, Shelly began to recount the story of the three fabulous days spent in Las Vegas while she had been in control of Amanda's body. Amanda had a textbook case of multiple-personality disorder, a fascinating and devastating response to trauma that has much to teach us about the nature of healing and the mind.

Some people who are severely abused or traumatized as children learn to survive in a particularly creative way. They dissociate from the terror, numbing themselves to what is happening and living in a fantasy—a set of images so realistic that the main character of their mental movie persists as an independent personality, or alter ego. For example, we know of a woman whose mother beat her when she was a child. She learned to "space out" when she heard her mother coming, and experienced herself playing outside. But someone, an alter ego or newly emergent personality, was left in control of her body to take the beating. That alter ego had unusual physical characteristics. It was an anesthetic personality that also had the capacity to encourage rapid wound healing. What a remarkable and creative response to pain!

Repetitive traumas may lead to several alter egos, which in some cases, may be totally unaware of one another. This is called multiple-personality disorder (MPD). There is currently heated professional debate over MPD. Although the disorder is listed in the psychiatric "bible," the DSM (Diagnosis and Statistical Manual) 4, some therapists believe that the disorder is overdiagnosed. Others believe that it doesn't exist at all. The latter group argues that MPD is a creation of well-meaning therapists who hypnotically implant alter egos by suggesting their existence. In just this fashion, false memories of abuse may sometimes be inadvertently implanted by therapists. But it is important not to throw out the baby with the bath water. Just as many cases of child abuse are true memories rather than false memories, many cases of MPD are also the result of severe trauma.

For example, can you imagine being a child in Bosnia? Perhaps one day a shell explodes in the schoolyard and you watch as your best friend's head explodes into a shower of bloody splinters. A week later your father is killed by a sniper on his way home from work. Next month you are gang-raped by soldiers who believe that because your religious beliefs are different from their own, you are less than human. Your little sister then becomes catatonic when yet another bomb blast rips through the neighborhood. And your mother is so very sad that she seems to have lost the will to live. When I think of the holocausts that so many children have endured, not only in war, but also in the inner city and in the confines of "family" life, I can only applaud the intelligence of the human spirit in its ability to form alternate lives in which we can preserve at least some semblance of sanity.

An adult multiple personality might have alter egos both older and younger than their chronological age. And amazingly, some of these personalities are physiologically distinct. One might need glasses, while others have normal vision. One might have a severe allergy that goes away when another alter ego emerges. There are cases in which one personality is addicted to a substance like heroin and only the addicted personality will undergo withdrawal. There are even cases where one personality has non-insulin dependent diabetes and the others are metabolically normal. What an amazing demonstration of the powers of the imagination to change the body! While Uncle Dick and his cheese phobia (mentioned in an earlier chapter) might seem mild by comparison, we're talking about the same principle—the power of the images in our mind to determine the state of the body.

Having spent nearly a decade of my life as a cancer cell biologist, I have wondered if it could be possible to have cancer in one personality but not others. The answer to that question isn't known, but I would guess that in a very small minority of cases such a thing would be possible. I have certainly heard reports of people who had multiple sclerosis in one personality that disappeared when another alter ego came out for any length of time. But, as amazing as these findings are for the body/mind, they also open up a window on the soul.

In the early 1960s, a psychiatrist by the name of Ralph Allison found that he could hypnotize multiple personalities and regress them to the time when each personality was split off as a result of some trauma. But there was always one personality that told a very different story from all the others. It did not report being formed at a traumatic time. Rather, it seemed to be an eternal, immortal essence. Independent of the patient's religious background, this personality said things such as, "I've been with this person before they were born, and I will remain with them after this body dies." It often characterized itself as a conduit for divine love or universal wisdom. Allison discovered that this core personality had remarkable insight, compassion, wit, and healing powers. If he could access it, this personality was often helpful in the therapy, with an uncanny knowledge of what the person needed in order to heal.

Allison dubbed this personality the Inner Self Helper, or ISH. Some of us might think of the ISH as our intuition, Higher Self, Divine Spark, or true Essence. When Miron and I first read about the ISH, it seemed strongly reminiscent of the core Self—the indwelling archetype of the Divine Essence that psychiatrist C. G. Jung had described. At about the same time that Jung described this core Self, with a capital *S* to distinguish it from our earthbound personality, or small self, the Italian psychiatrist Roberto Assagioli also described a spiritual essence, called Self, at the core of every person.

Assagioli's work reminded us of the Buddhist image of the Rigpa (one's own true nature or Higher Self), as a sun that is always shining, although for most of us it is obscured by clouds. These clouds comprise the collection of opinions, beliefs, and behaviors that we develop as children to keep us safe in the world. They represent the hypnotic trance in which we live our lives. Assagioli calls these clouds *subpersonalities*. Spiritual systems such as *A Course in Miracles* describe these fear-based beliefs as *the ego*. The ego in this sense is different from its usage in standard psychological parlance as a strong and healthy sense of self.

Since we all have an array of subpersonalities, we're all a little bit like multiple personalities. Sometimes I'm in my writer or teacher subpersonality, and that can be very creative and life affirming. But if my entire sense of self was wrapped up in being a teacher, and then I retired, I might find myself seriously depressed, as do many retired people. Sometimes a woman is overidentified with the mother subpersonality and feels worthless and despondent when her children leave home. Subpersonalities are creative when we realize that they are part of our wholeness. They become traps when we believe that any one of them is the entire measure of who we are.

Some subpersonalities are obvious. I can recognize my teacher, mother, and lover roles. The images that play in my mind, the emotions I experience, and the feelings in my body are very different when I'm feeling the expansive exuberance of love as opposed to when I'm trapped in my fear-based martyr, rescuer, victim, or critic subpersonalities. Long experience has demonstrated that my rare migraine headaches usually occur when I've lost my sense of openness to the possibilities of the moment and am stuck in the angry, hurt, limiting images of the victim.

A remarkable woman by the name of Alice Hopper Epstein wrote a book called *Mind, Fantasy and Healing* about working with her subpersonalities and experiencing a spontaneous remission from kidney cancer. Her story was featured on the inspiring six-part series, *Exploring the Heart of Healing*, telecast on Turner Broadcasting in 1993 and 1994. The series was produced by the Institute of Noetic Sciences, a membership organization dedicated to the exploration of healing and human consciousness, from which you can order the videotapes. (Information about the Institute of Noetic Sciences can be found in the Resources section of the Appendix.)

Alice, as she tells her story, was working unhappily on a doctorate in sociology when the cancer was diagnosed. Like many of us strivers and achievers, she was hoping that a doctorate would finally make her feel worthy and lovable. For, although she was surrounded by people who really cared, she described herself as unable to take in and experience their love. As she talked about her feelings of worthlessness and inability to experience joy, I felt her pain deeply because it was so reminiscent of my own in earlier times.

When the cancer was discovered, it had already metastasized to her lungs. The situation was dire. There was no proven treatment for metastatic kidney cancer, and Alice's only medical hope was an experimental trial of interferon. Since interferon treatment could not start right away, Alice and her husband, Seymour Epstein, at that time a professor of psychology at the University of Massachusetts, decided to try a no-holds-barred psychological approach to healing. They chose to work with a psychosynthesis therapist. Alice soon discovered a child subpersonality—a five-year old she called Mickey—who seemed bent on self-destruction. Psychosynthesis utilizes very powerful exercises of imagination to heal subpersonalities such as Mickey and bring forth the wisdom that is latent within every wound. Alice completely gave herself over to this healing work.

When it was time to begin the experimental interferon treatment, Alice's x-rays showed that the lung tumors had shrunk substantially! Since her condition was improving, she decided to decline the interferon and continue with the psychosynthesis. Over a period of months, the cancers continued to shrink. Alice and her husband were able to track striking parallels between breakthroughs in the psychosynthesis work and regression of the tumors. Over a decade later, Alice is cancer free. Her life is also healed. Able to give and receive love, she radiates joy and a quiet peacefulness.

While stories such as Alice's are inspiring, they might also tempt us to oversimplify the link between cancer and the mind. Although Alice's tumors seemed clearly related to the subpersonality Mickey, such a one-to-one correspondence is probably quite rare. When I asked Alice's opinion about this phenomenon, she readily agreed. She theorizes that probably only a few percent of cancers are as closely tied to the set of beliefs, images, and behaviors that define personality, as hers was. But even if Alice's cancer had not been cured, her quality of life would still have been dramatically improved through the psychological healing work. As we've said before, the measure of our success is not in the length of life, but in our capacity to give and receive love.

In a spiritual sense, healing is the process of harvesting the teachings from our wounds. In the process, we develop true self-respect and the ability to see others with the same respect. This compassionate awareness leaves us open to the creative possibilities in all situations. When the clouds of ego clear away, we express the compassion and joy that really are our own true nature or Higher Self.

In the past year, we have heard a wonderful quote attributed to Ram Dass, Wayne Dyer, Deepak Chopra, and a nameless Catholic priest, which is: *"We are not human beings having a spiritual experience. We are spiritual beings having a human experience."* When this paradigm shift really sinks into our cells, we begin the process of awakening from the dream of our wounds to the power of the wisdom we gain in their healing.

CHAPTER EIGHTEEN

EMOTIONAL HEALING

I can still remember giving my first lecture to 150 medical students, not to mention the fearsome back row of faculty members who, I was sure, were keeping track of all my errors. It was terrifying. But after three or four more lectures, I gradually got accustomed to teaching. Miron, however, had a very different experience. As he readily admits, he used to be one of the worst lecturers of all time because he became literally sick with panic every time he had to speak. Unlike me, he didn't adapt to the situation.

While fear of public speaking is very common, Miron's fear was exaggerated, almost incapacitating. I taught him basic meditation and breathing exercises, which helped to some degree. At least he could sleep the night before, manage his stomach cramps, and give his lectures. But, as Miron says, these lectures were mediocre at best and certainly didn't reflect his mastery of the subject matter. For a long time, he rationalized his poor lecture performance by blaming the students—they were just "spoiled rich kids" eager to judge him. He also blamed the system of medical education since it valued research more than teaching and provided little or nothing in the way of teacher education. Miron's choice to manage his anxieties by blaming others left him playing the role of the victim.

One day during this period, a friend of ours called. He was a Boston police detective and hypnotist whose job it was to hypnotize victims of crimes in the hopes of getting information that would help apprehend the perpetrator. Like us, "Dave" had an avid interest in healing, healers, and the power of the mind. He told Miron about a healing service that was held one Sunday each month at the Mission Hill Church in Boston. Following some prayers and a brief introduction, the priest blessed people with holy water. Some of them actually fell backward into a swoon, and many testified to physical or emotional healings. Although Dave hadn't gone to the church for a physical healing, he was surprised when a chronically ingrown toenail healed a week later.

Miron was intrigued by the description of the healing service, so we decided to "check it out." The Mission Hill Church is located in a once-elegant section of Boston, bordering the dangerous ghetto area called Roxbury, which was once a neighborhood of gorgeous old mansions and townhouses. An island of splendor in a sea of decay, the church had managed to maintain the beauty of that former era. Dedicated to Mary, as are many of the great European cathedrals, it was filled with magnificent stained glass, sculpture, and medieval friezes. Clouds of sweet incense curled toward a ceiling that seemed only slightly less ornate than that of the Sistine Chapel. Rows of angels and beautifully carved confessionals lined the walls.

The opulence of the church prepared me mentally for a charismatic preacher whose energy would fill the impressive cathedral. Instead, we found Father MacDonough to be a quiet, humble man without a big personality. There was no fanfare to begin the service, just some prayers and a few songs by the community choir. Several hundred people, including a number of children, sat patiently in the pews. The priest then invited anyone who needed healing to come up to the rail of the sanctuary to be blessed. Miron and I watched from our seats. I was amazed when some people fell over backwards as they were blessed. "Mass hypnosis," I thought, feeling the same resistance arising in me that I had felt as a nine-year-old during the birthday party with the hypnotist. Two big men walked behind the row of supplicants catching those who fell, placing them gently on the cool marble floor. No way was I going to fall over!

After a few minutes, Miron and I lined up to take our turns. As a drop of holy water touched my face, an incredible peace spread throughout my body, a peace so deep that my muscles just gave way. Two strong arms caught me as I sank down into an ocean of bliss. I looked up from the floor to see Miron grinning down at me. After a few minutes, my muscles recovered and I walked back to the pew to find that Miron had had a different, but equally remarkable, response to the blessing. He was weeping from the depths of his soul. In the decade or more that we'd been married, I had never seen him cry. His tears flowed throughout the remainder of the service.

When we emerged from the dark womb of the church into the bright light of day, I asked Miron why he'd been crying. Oddly enough, he didn't have a clue. Just as I had been simply overwhelmed with peace, he had been overcome by grief. As the weeks passed, he still couldn't figure out what had happened. So when the Sunday of the healing service came on the following month, he suggested that we return to the church with a few friends. This time he began to cry from the moment he set foot in the church to the moment we left, nearly two hours later. People were sending us tissues from several rows away.

This time we were determined to figure out what the tears were about, so I guided him in the mirror exercise described in detail in my book about emotional healing, *Guilt Is the Teacher, Love Is the Lesson*. He got comfortable and shifted into belly breathing, accessing the place of inner wisdom where the mind begins to quiet. Then he visualized the number three, and let the three melt into a two, the two into a one, and the one into a zero. Then he let the zero elongate into an oval mirror and asked to be shown a scene that related to why he was crying in the church.

Immediately, he flashed on a scene from his childhood. He was about seven and had recently emigrated to America following the end of World War II. His parents had trekked across Europe on foot, fleeing from their Russian oppressors. Captured by the Gestapo, they were fortunate that their stay in a concentration camp only lasted a few months, especially since Miron's mother was pregnant. After Miron's birth, they slowly made their way to safety in the American sector of Germany, their path often perilously close to the front lines where bombs and shells were exploding. His parents were survivors, arriving at Ellis Island with a boatload of seasick refugees, a six-year-old boy, and five dollars to start a new life. Once in New York, Miron used to joke wryly, his life took a major turn for the worse when his parents sent him to Catholic school.

The scene he saw in the mirror was of himself, alone in the family's apartment, crying in bitter frustration and anguish, banging his knee against the wall. It was evening. His mother was out learning English, and his father was at work in a factory. Miron wasn't afraid of being alone, so at first he didn't remember what the problem was. So, he asked the mirror again. The next scene that appeared was of his first-grade parochial school classroom. The teaching nun had asked him to come up front and read. He stood there filled with shame, his little hands shaking, because he didn't speak a single word of English. The nun stormed up, pulled out his hand, and beat him with a ruler. Several months later, she sent him to be evaluated for mental retardation. Somehow, in the midst of a massive period of immigration, it had escaped her that this lonely little boy spoke only Ukrainian.

No wonder Miron had an aversion to speaking in front of groups! And no wonder his grief had been compounded by a healing service in a Catholic church. The time had come to heal a painful memory that not only limited Miron's ability to teach, but also limited his ability to connect with God. For most of his life, Miron had believed that God was a sorry excuse for persecution in the name of righteousness. After all, when religion teaches fear instead of love, what else can a child be expected to think?

Once Miron became aware of the childhood trauma he had endured, the next step was to heal his wounds. From the perspective of his adult self, he was able to imagine holding his seven-year-old self and reassuring him that he was not to blame. Patiently explaining the truth of what had happened and giving the child the chance to express his emotions, Miron lovingly healed the memory—which included forgiving the nun. Whenever I heal my own memories, or those of clients, I always finish the process by enclosing the scene in a bubble of light and sending it back to the Universe.

The retrieval of the memory clarified some basic, life-guiding decisions that Miron had made as a child. Such decisions are not conscious choices. They are unconscious mechanisms of survival. To protect himself from abuse by authority figures such as the nun, he had developed an authoritarian, judgmental part of his own nature. If that part of him could have talked to the nun, perhaps it might have said, "I'm tough and you can't get me. Besides, I'm just like you. I bet you respect me now." There was also a part of him that found safety in being a victim because he could get love from his parents, who wanted to soothe his hurts. Can you recognize these two parts of Miron in his interactions with the medical students?

In psychosynthesis terms, Miron's Victim subpersonality was in cahoots with his Judge. The Judge protected the Victim, and the Victim received sympathy, a poor substitute for love and respect, but at least a reassurance that he was cared for. When we are children, our world view is shaped by the need for love. How can we act, what can we say, to ensure the continual bestowal of love by our primary caretakers? Abandonment means psychological, if not physical, death to a child. Love is as critical to survival as food and shelter. In the process of adapting to our home, school, and cultural situations, we develop a whole system of subpersonalities similar to Miron's. These subpersonalities can be compared to masks that hide our true nature even from ourselves. Until we heal the wounds that formed them, we tend to compulsively act out the old stories from childhood with new people. Our true creativity and power cannot shine forth.

The change in Miron after healing these subpersonalities was profound. He began to see his students as people just like him, with their own fears and insecurities. He noticed how they worried about absorbing the enormous amount of subject matter in their courses. Would they flunk out? Could they make it as physicians? For the first time, he saw the students as people rather than as oppressors. On the day that his heart broke open in church, compassion began to flow. Emotional healing had kept his heart open, and he could finally empathize with the students' pain because he had lovingly faced his own.

Miron also opened his heart to his parents. His father, Dimitri, had been very distant as Miron grew up, and he felt as if they hardly knew one another. So, Miron decided to drive to upper New York State where his parents lived to try to make a heart-to-heart connection with his father. The entire five-hour drive from Boston was spent trying to figure out how to open up a meaningful conversation. He finally decided to make the simple request: "Tell me about your childhood."

Miron's father had lived through a holocaust that is rarely spoken of, the terrible starvation that Stalin inflicted on the Ukrainian people, in which more than seven million people perished. As an adolescent, Dimitri had watched many of his childhood friends wither away and finally die. A mother in his village, crazed from grief and hunger, actually ate her own daughter. Dimitri and his mother managed to survive only because he had the foresight to hide grain in numerous gourds and hang them in trees all over the countryside. In addition, his mother still had a cow. He spoke of how the neighbor's children would line up, waiting for the daily glass of milk that was all the nourishment some of them had.

Dimitri cried as he remembered one little girl spilling the milk down her dress because she had become too weak to even drink. No wonder he'd been so distant all his life—depressed and stuck in the memories of his own private hell. As Miron listened to the story, the distance he had felt from his father melted away. Anger and hurt were replaced by love and understanding. There was no question of forgiving his father, because it was clear that he had done the best he could. Miron's healing deepened while listening to his father's story, and his father was also healed when he saw the respect and love that shone from his son's eyes.

As a result of these months of healing, Miron finally overcame his fear of public speaking. When he put down his Victim and Judge masks, he was at last free to become himself. He ended up winning Tufts Medical School's outstanding teacher award for four years in a row until he finally left academia. As you might imagine, his healing has changed our home life, too. The tendency to blame, which is one of the greatest toxins in a relationship, is practically nonexistent now. And the authoritarian, distant father of our children's youth has grown into a loving, supportive parent. One of the greatest joys we've both had in our long marriage is the continual deepening of our love for one another and our children as both of us have continued to heal.

Since relatively few of us were loved unconditionally as children, we can do only marginally better with our own kids. This is the meaning of the biblical statement that the sins of the father are visited on the children. Sin, after all, simply means separation. When we are separated from love, we become hypnotized by fear. Then we naturally teach fear rather than love because it is all we know. Every mask we put on, every subpersonality that we mistake for who we really are, is simply an expression of the fear that we are not lovable. Each person who heals him- or herself of this illusion helps break the chain of fear that has extended back in a long progression through our families and throughout our world.

Stop for a minute and think of two or three masks that you learned to wear as a child. What are they? Can you understand how they sometimes get in the way of your ability to love and create? Are you ready to heal them and claim the wisdom in your wounds?

Each of our subpersonalities is a *samskara*, an imprint on our souls, which is comfortably worn with use and which we will continue to live from until we consciously become aware of the pattern and choose to heal it. When we do, each subpersonality will become a jewel in our crown of wisdom. For example, behind the mask of the Victim lies the gift of a compassionate heart. Once we have suffered and healed, we have particular empathy for the suffering of others. Behind the mask of the Perfectionist lies a deep appreciation for beauty and balance. The healed Judge becomes a fine discriminator, capable of acknowledging the unique gifts of every person.

Someone at a workshop once asked Miron what the jewel in the healed Martyr was. He had to stop and think. The Martyr is certainly one of my subpersonalities, but it isn't one of his. "The healer Martyr," he replied, "is a person who can suffer with dignity and grace because suffering is inevitable, but misery is optional!" I laughed, recalling my mother, who would sweat for days in a hot kitchen preparing the holiday meal, and then refuse to sit down and eat with us. She believed she had to serve and complain. In this role, she found some worthiness. Having been tutored in martyrdom from an early age, I can say that, for me, worthiness is the jewel of the Martyr. As part of my healing, I've learned to feel good about my being, not about a show of doing in which I give my life force away.

There are as many ways to heal old emotional wounds as there are schools of psychotherapy. As with meditation, different methods are suitable for different people. One caution, however, lies in making any process of healing your primary identity. This is just putting on one more mask to buy love. While 12-step programs have served to heal many millions of people, a few get addicted to their program and become professional 12-steppers. They are Sue or Sam, the Recovering Alcoholic. When you introduce yourself to people outside a recovery program as an adult child of an alcoholic or as an incest survivor, you have seriously limited your being. You are much greater than the sum of your wounds, no matter how grievous they might have been. (A wonderful metaphysically oriented book that deals with this very subject is *Your Companion to 12 Step Recovery*, by Robert Odom, published by Hay House.)

Similarly, some people get stuck in healing their inner child to the point where they elevate it to the status of brat-in-residence. Miron and our older son Justin once went to a men's group led by the poet and writer Robert Bly. One of the men in the group began to wax eloquent about the warm and wonderful relationship he had with his inner child, how he took him fishing and fathered him. Bly, in his endearingly blunt manner, yelled, "Well, then it's time to kill the little son-of-a-bitch now, isn't it?" What he meant was that, ultimately, healing is a letting-go, not a hanging-on. We need to heal our wounded inner children and let them grow up into emotionally mature, wise adults rather than coddling them for a lifetime.

Each stage of our life is marked by death and birth. Just as our infant self dies to become a child, our child self must die to achieve adulthood. Emotional healing is a series of deaths and rebirths. Every time we put fear to death, we are reborn to a deeper ability to love.

CHAPTER NINETEEN

TAKING OFF THE MASK AND FINDING THE HIGHER SELF

Perhaps you've heard the joke that a codependent is a person who, at the moment of death, sees someone else's life flash in front of their eyes! The process of healing entails becoming ourselves by taking off the masks we have worn to please others. Now that you know the story of how Miron discovered and healed two masks that were preventing him from being himself, we'd like to introduce you to a powerful exercise we have used for years to heal sub-personalities.

I originally adapted this exercise from a healing meditation that we learned from therapist Robin Casarjian. She, in turn, had adapted it from a psychosynthesis exercise. Oftentimes, the best results occur when you have the fewest expectations. Sometimes nothing happens at all in these healing meditations, which we call inner-wisdom exercises, except that you notice your own fidgety mind. Other times you may get some insight, but it is just an extension of something you already knew. Sometimes, of course, a tremendous breakthrough occurs. But whether or not healing seems to flow directly from the exercise, if you do it with a sincere desire for growth, your intention itself is a powerful prayer that will bring healing help to you.

The first few times you try this exercise, it's a good idea to have a supportive person available to talk with afterwards. A wonderful way to work with this meditation is to tape it, using a soft musical background, and then listen to it with a friend or partner. We've found that the best way to debrief afterwards is for each person to take as long as they need to tell about their experience *without interruption*. The other person sits and listens with interest and respect. After one person has finished, the other person has a turn. Only after both stories have been told do you have a discussion. In this way, both of you get the chance to talk without the other person interrupting with interpretations or advice which, though well intended, can short-circuit your learning. One outcome of such an exercise is that you may discover deep-seated issues that require a professional listener, a therapist, to facilitate your healing.

I must have done this exercise with the mask I call the Judge at least ten times, and I've acquired a little bit more insight on each occasion. The last time I tried it, the Judge had changed its form entirely from the banshee-like creature it had once been into an old and trusted friend. I've learned a lot from this part of myself. The masks that used to bother me most were the Judge, the Complainer, the Control Freak, the Victim, and the Rescuer. Some of the most common masks people work with are the Perfectionist, the Martyr, the Judge, the Glamour Girl, the Macho Man, the People-Pleaser, the Victim, the Aggressor, the Enforcer, the Genius, the Dope, the Rebel, and the Saint. The variations are endless.

The best clues to show you when you're wearing a mask is that other people may be reacting poorly toward you, or you may be feeling uncomfortable—that is, tense, anxious, self-conscious, irritable, or afraid. Remember that each one of these masks was formed to protect you from the loss of love, which means that they are organized around fear. If you are in your authentic, or Higher Self, you generally feel confident, open-hearted, and loving. So, one way to deepen your awareness of the masks you wear is to pay attention to things that upset you. For example, did you ever react to something that someone said or to some circumstance in an irrational way, or in a manner that was entirely out of proportion to the situation? Sometimes the slightest remark leaves us feeling mortally wounded, full of self-righteousness or seething with rage.

Before you choose a time to try the emotional healing exercise below, *make sure to have a specific mask in mind*. The purpose of this exercise is to become more aware of the mask you chose and to realize some of the ways in which it has been truly helpful to you and some of the ways in which it has limited you. The mask is a real, living part of your psyche, and like all living things, it needs your respect and love. You will have a chance to make a friend and ally of this part of yourself and to use its gifts in the service of your Higher Self rather than in service of the ego and its fears.

TAKING OFF THE MASK AND FINDING THE HIGHER SELF

Take a good stretch, and when you're ready, close your eyes...

Begin to pay attention to your breathing, noticing its rhythm....The way your belly rises on the inbreath....And how you relax and let go on the outbreath....

Now, in your mind's eye, imagine that you are coming to a door....What does it look like? How does it feel when you touch it? In just a moment you can open the door and find one of your masks behind it, a part of yourself that you would like to know better, to understand, help, and be enriched by....

Open the door now and meet this mask....It may be a person, an image, an animal, or a kind of thought....If the door seems stuck or nothing seems to appear, what would you meet if the door did open or something did appear? How does your mask appear to you?

Take this part of yourself and go to your innermost place of wisdom, imagining that sacred center as a summer meadow on a sunlit day....Spend a moment appreciating the lushness of the grass, trees, and flowers that shine inwardly with a living light...the fragrances...the colors...the warmth of the sun....The more you open to the beauty, the more you can feel the sacred presence of your own Higher Self and the Beings of Light who are always ready to come to your aid.

Feel the sunlight shining down upon you and washing over you....Feel it running through you, filling you with vitality, clarity, and compassion....Feel it filling your heart and emerging through your eyes....

Now, look at your mask, also bathed in light....The light pouring over it and shining out through it....Communicate from the deepest level of your being your intent to know, love, and understand this aspect of yourself....

Now, ask this part of yourself, "How are you trying to help me?" Listen carefully for the answers....Ask when during your life it came into being....

Thank your mask for the help it has given you....

Explain carefully how its attempts to help sometimes hurt you, especially when they come from old fears....

Ask it to cooperate with you in operating out of its highest wisdom, in service to your Higher Self....

Ask how you can help it operate out of its highest potential....Then imagine a scene of how this would appear in your life....

Take a moment and finish your conversation in any way you need to....

Feel the warm light shining down upon both of you....If any fear remains, allow it to dry up in the sunlight and blow into the field where its dust can nourish the flowers....

Take the beautiful, loving being that was the core of the mask all along, and tuck it into your heart....

Rest in the peace, love, and wisdom of your Higher Self....and know that your healing is also a healing for the world soul.

When you are ready, take a deep breath and a stretch, coming back at your own pace...taking your time until you feel ready to open your eyes.

CHAPTER TWENTY

FORGIVENESS AND COMPASSION

My mother, martyr though she may have been, was one of the funniest people I've ever known. Sometimes I fantasize seeing her in a nightclub like the intergalactic bar in the movie *Star Wars*, smoking a cigarette and tossing off one-liners about highly amusing earthlings she has known. The morning before she died, the doctor sent her down to the nuclear medicine department in the hospital so that they could pinpoint the location of internal bleeding that marked the last stage of her long illness, what Miron called *apetrolonemia,* or running out of gas.

Most of the family was gathered in her seventh-floor room that windy March day, waiting to say their final goodbyes. Hours passed, and she was still missing somewhere in the bowels of the hospital basement where the big machinery was housed. Since I'd worked in that same hospital for many years, the family sent me down to retrieve her. We were really concerned that she might die on a stretcher in some lonely corridor and that we wouldn't be there when she needed us most. I marched resolutely down to nuclear medicine in the hopes that they would unhand her, but I also knew how hard it is to buck hospital policy.

I gathered my courage and barged into the room where she was being held, yet to be tested. I confronted the doctor, explaining that six hours was a long wait under these circumstances. He explained impatiently that she had to stay for the test because it was essential to have a diagnosis for the bleeding. My mother, who had been lying on her stretcher literally at death's door, piped up, "Diagnosis? All you want is a diagnosis? I'm dying. That's your diagnosis." And you know, he couldn't argue with her logic, so soon we were on our way back to her room.

During that short elevator ride, we accomplished the work of a lifetime. Mom, who was not a woman to discuss emotions, looked up at me with the innocent eyes of a child, and said simply, "I've made a lot of mistakes. Will you forgive me?" My heart just melted, and all the difficulties we'd had over a lifetime vanished in the magic of that moment. Then I thought about all the times I'd been angry with her, impatient, judgmental, or just plain absent. I so wished it had been different. I wished we could have been friends. With my heart in my throat, I asked her to forgive me. We sealed the deal with a touch of the fingers and a look in the eyes. How very precious those few moments were.

There is a saying in *A Course in Miracles* that "the holiest ground is where an ancient hatred has become a present love." Difficult circumstances and negative emotions are meant to be the raw materials for soul growth. Our most problematic relationships represent holy ground being tilled. When I tell the story of that moment of forgiveness that mother and I shared, people's eyes often get teary. For some, the tears are a deep recognition of the sacred. For others they are an expression of grief for forgiveness not yet realized.

If we're willing to do the work of emotional healing, those very people and circumstances that injured us can turn out to be the transformers through which we find the richness of our humanity. Our own philosophy is very resonant with that of *A Course in Miracles,* which simplifies healing: *Make peace of mind your only goal and forgiveness your only function.* Forgiveness, indeed, is the way to peace of mind.

The very word *forgiveness*, though, lends itself to weighty misunderstandings. For some of us it conjures up the notion of copping out by turning the other cheek and allowing another person to get away with something. That's not forgiveness at all. In the words of Bob Hoffman, the founder of a remarkable psychospiritual healing program called The Hoffman Quadrinity Process, that's "putting whipped cream on top of garbage." In *Guilt Is the Teacher, Love Is the Lesson,* I outline a process of forgiveness that consists of several steps. First comes a period of grieving for what has been lost. Second comes anger about the loss. The eventual acceptance of one's loss is the third step. What is done is done. We might as well make lemonade out of lemons by learning something that will strengthen us. Lemonade is the fourth step, a paradigm shift in which we are able to find some good, some meaning, in our difficulty.

You might have noticed that nowhere in the previous paragraph did I actually mention changing your feelings toward the person who hurt you. When steps one through four are completed, feelings about the other person naturally and organically change. Without making a particular point of it, you may come to understand the circumstances that led to their actions and feel compassion, as Miron did for his father. But as compassionate as we may feel, forgiveness has no behavioral strings attached—ours or theirs. We may forgive a person and still call the police. We may forgive a person and choose never to see them again because their hurtful behavior is unlikely to change. Forgiveness is our own responsibility and has nothing to do with apologies or amends on the part of the other, as nice as these might be.

A woman we know who was the survivor of a brutal rape by her uncle defined forgiveness as "freedomness." Her uncle had been dead for years, but she was still bound to him by her hatred. Forgiveness finally set her free. Prior to forgiveness, we are indeed bound to the object of our hate. Resentment occupies our thoughts and poisons our body/mind. It is a powerful adversary that keeps us from being fully present in the moment. As long as we are shackled by hatred or judgment, we cannot claim the true power of our mind to heal. We are prisoners of the past.

Stop and reflect for a minute. *Are you currently holding a grudge against anyone? If so, ask yourself what good that grudge does for you. Is it making you stronger, wiser, more peaceful, or more powerful? How are you feeling right now when you think of your resentment? Is this how you really want to feel? Is it a conscious choice?*

When we have been victimized, we sometimes mistake anger for power. This emotional misunderstanding escalates the cycle of violence when victims of crime grow up to be perpetrators. Most of the men and women in our prison system were abused as children. Until they learn how to forgive both their abusers and themselves, our jails will remain houses of detention rather than places of healing. Our good friend and colleague Robin Casarjian, author of *Forgiveness: A Bold Choice for a Peaceful Heart*, has been working in the Massachusetts prison system for many years. She is writing a book called *Houses of Healing*, drawing on the first-hand transformations she has witnessed in men and women who have committed themselves to the healing programs she facilitates.

Robin created the Lionheart Foundation, a nonprofit agency, to distribute *Houses of Healing*, with accompanying audiotapes and videotapes, free to every prison in the United States. (You can find information about how to support this important project in the Resources section of the Appendix.) Many of the prisoners Robin has worked with have finally been able to take responsibility for their crimes after healing the wounds of their own childhood. We can't open our hearts to others unless they are first open to ourselves. Her program of healing childhood wounds, understanding the emotions, and practicing forgiveness toward self and others is the only thing we can imagine that truly has the power to stop the escalating cycle of violence in our country.

Once we, like the men and women Robin works with, realize that anger is a prison and not a power, we are on the road to a new way of living. The Buddha compared anger to a hot coal that we pick up, intending to throw at someone else, only to be burned ourselves. When you can get an hour or two to yourself, sit down with a pad of paper or your journal and think back through your life to each person who hurt you. Make a list of them. Then ask yourself whether you're still hurt and angry or whether you've healed. Ask yourself what you learned from each person, and write that information down next to their name. Even the most egregious injury produces a pearl of wisdom.

However, if you find that there are some people whom you can't even begin to forgive, perhaps you would be willing to tell the story of what happened to someone you trust—not as an advertisement for your hurt, but as a way to get insight on step four—what you can learn from the situation. If you still feel hurt and anger, you may want to seek professional help. Letting go of regrets and resentments is the cornerstone of achieving peace of mind. An interviewer once asked who had taught me most about life. I mentally ran down the list of people who had sustained me as a child: teachers, friends, spiritual mentors, and loved ones. Remarkably, the "enemies" who had wounded me most were my greatest teachers and healers.

When the Dalai Lama is asked about his feelings toward the Chinese, who carried out a hideous holocaust in Tibet during the 1950s, he always teaches forgiveness. In one interview, he commented on the compassion he felt for people who exhibited such pain and ignorance—qualities that would allow them to act so unconsciously toward others. As he spoke, the video flashed back to scenes of the Chinese raping Tibetan nuns, burning down monasteries, and decimating the land. I could feel anger rising within me at the same time the Dalai Lama smiled and radiated his uniquely peaceful presence. He continued his teachings on forgiveness by mentioning that he practiced a form of meditation in which he took on the pain of the Chinese and returned his peace and happiness to them. I don't know whether I would be capable of such altruism in the same circumstance, but this philosophy has certainly helped me release lesser hurts. The name of this ancient forgiveness meditation is *tonglen*, the meditation of giving and receiving.

Unbeknownst to either of us, my mother unconsciously practiced tonglen with me. When I was sick, either as a child or as an adult, she would sincerely wish that she could take on my sickness and give me her health. This is another way to look at *for give ness*. Love is *for giving* away. When we do that, giving the best in ourselves to another, we feel the love and receive healing ourselves. Old legend actually credits tonglen with the power to heal the practitioner of leprosy and even cancer.

The basic exchange in tonglen is energetic, accomplished by an exercise of creative imagination. You bring another person to mind and imagine their pain, illness, or ignorance as a black smoke around their heart. Inhaling their smoke into your own heart, you imagine that it neutralizes your own smokescreen, revealing the sun in your heart. You then exhale the sun—the light, love, and peace of your own true nature—into the other person's heart. You continue this practice for several breaths until it feels complete.

Even though I'm an ex-smoker, breathing in the smoke of other people's pain feels fine to me. Every so often in a workshop, however, someone is too bothered by the image of the smoke to practice tonglen. If this is true for you, just imagine the smoke as dark clouds surrounding the other person's heart, and breathe in the clouds. Somehow I don't think that the ancient Tibetan lamas would mind. One's intention is far more powerful than specific details.

The practice of tonglen is reminiscent of the lovingkindness meditation we learned in Chapter 15. We do it first for ourselves, then for loved ones, next for "enemies," and finally for all beings. Jesus taught forgiveness in much the same way when he said, "Love the Lord thy God with all thy heart, with all thy soul and with all thy mind, and love thy neighbor as thyself." The first stage in the practice of compassion and forgiveness is to feel it for ourselves. If there is no room in our heart for us, how can we have anything of value to give anyone else?

Once you have learned tonglen, which we will teach at the end of this chapter, you can use it in real-life situations to practice a forgiving attitude—one of nonjudgment. It is also an excellent way to transform negative emotions into love.

Let me give you an example. Walking around bookstores can sometimes be hard for me. The book you have in your hand is my sixth. I've poured my whole heart and mind into each book, and I believe that every one is uniquely helpful. So, naturally, it hurts when bookstores don't carry them.

When I first enter a bookstore, I often browse nonchalantly, then I gradually progress to checking the health, psychology, and spirituality shelves where my books might be. When I don't find them, I sometimes feel dejected. All that work for nothing. Then I might look around and see a tall stack of the latest self-help book and mumble something like, "Ugh. What a superficial, stupid book. She tells people what they want to hear, not what they need to heal. Who buys all this junk?!" Soon I'm depressed, envious, greedy, and angry.

A few letting-go breaths later, I usually remember that I have a choice. I can stew in my misery or I can let go of it. But with tonglen, I can do something even better. I can transform the emotional misery and use its inherent energy for spiritual growth. Once you are used to doing tonglen with your eyes closed, it is easy to do a short form with your eyes open. Pretending that I'm thumbing through a book, I imagine that I can see myself as if looking into a mirror. I inhale the black smoke of envy, depression, greed, and anger, feel it parting the clouds around my heart, and exhale love back at myself. After four or five breaths, not only have I regained sanity, I actually feel much better than before.

Tonglen also works well when you catch yourself judging some other person. Years ago I attended a lecture by Ram Dass in which he pointed out that our judgments about others are projections about what we don't like in ourselves. Whenever we catch ourselves in the midst of such a projection, he recommends saying, "And I am that, too." While I have found this method very helpful in making me aware of such projections, tonglen can actually transform them. Whether I'm talking to someone, thinking about someone, or walking down the street judging a complete stranger, tonglen works wonders. I breathe in the smoke from around their heart (really from around my own) and breathe back the respect and love of my own Higher Self. Excellent instructions for tonglen can be found in Sogyal Rinpoche's *Tibetan Book of Living and Dying*.

Tonglen is also very useful when watching the news or hearing of a disaster anywhere in the world. Rather than feeling overwhelmed by sadness, or hardening our hearts and numbing out, tonglen is a way of saying an immediate prayer for transformation. For example, I was watching a newsclip from Bosnia in late 1993. A distraught mother was bending over the dead body of her only son, keening with sorrow. The dead boy looked even younger than our own sons, and my heart just broke. While continuing to watch the clip, I breathed in the pain of this mother and breathed back the love and peace in my own heart both to her and to her child. Sogyal Rinpoche recommends that if you have cancer or AIDS or any illness, you might do tonglen for all the other people with the same problem. Health-care professionals can do tonglen for their patients, and we can all do it for one another. When Sogyal Rinpoche was asked whether you could hurt yourself by breathing in another person's illness, he laughed and replied, "The only thing you can hurt is your ego!" Nonetheless, if doing tonglen for someone feels wrong for you, don't do it. A recovering codependent asked me a somewhat similar question. Isn't tonglen just another way of sponging up other people's pain, she wondered—a habit she was trying to get out of? In fact, tonglen is just the opposite. Instead of taking on someone else's pain, you are using their pain to transform your own suffering.

TONGLEN:
The Meditation of Forgiveness and Compassion

Close your eyes and take a stretch and a few letting-go breaths....Begin to notice the flow of your breathing, allowing your body to relax and your mind to come to rest....

Imagine a Great Star of Light above your head, and feel it washing over you like a waterfall and running through you like a river runs through the sand at its bottom....Allow it to carry away any fatigue, pain, illness, or ignorance....See these wash through the bottom of your feet into the earth for transformation. As you are washed clean, notice that the light within your heart begins to shine very brightly....

Now imagine yourself as a child, choosing whatever age seems most relevant to you at this time....You, better than anyone, know the pain in your heart at that time. Breathe it in as a black smoke (or dark clouds), and breathe out the light in your heart to yourself....

Imagine yourself as you are right now, as if you could see yourself in a mirror. See whatever pain or illness you have as a black smoke around your heart. Inhale the smoke and exhale the light of your Higher Self....Fill your heart with light....

Bring to mind a person that you love....Think about the pain or illness that might be in their heart....Inhale that pain as a black smoke, and exhale the light of your own true nature back into their heart.

Bring to mind someone whom you are ready to forgive. Imagine them in as much detail as you can. Imagine their pain, illness, or illusion as a black smoke around their heart....Breathe in the smoke, and breathe back the light of your own true nature into their heart.

Think of someplace in the world where there is suffering. If possible, bring a specific example of that suffering to mind—a starving child, a grieving parent....Breathe in the pain of that suffering as a black smoke, and let it part the clouds of darkness around your own heart. Breathe out the light of your Higher Self.

End with a prayer or a short period of mindful meditation. You may also want to dedicate the fruits of this meditation to alleviate the suffering of all beings:

> *May all beings be happy.*
> *May all be free from suffering.*
> *May all know the beauty of*
> *their own true nature.*
> *May all beings be healed.*

CHAPTER TWENTY-ONE

A SCIENTIST MEETS THE ANGELS:
Help from Other Realms

One day late in the fall of 1988, I was standing in line at a ticket counter at Boston's Logan Airport, waiting to check in for a business trip. When my turn came, the ticket agent was unusually courteous and helpful, offering to move me to a more comfortable seat. I commented on her kindness, particularly noteworthy because of the long line queued up in back of me. Without missing a beat, she replied that if she were not kind to everyone she would hear about it from her spirit guides that night! I held my breath for a moment, thinking, "Shall I follow up on this or not—the line is really long."

Throwing caution to the winds, I asked, "Do you meditate to get in touch with your guides?" Still tapping away at her computer, she answered matter-of-factly, "No, I've always been able to talk with them. I'm psychic, and so is my mother." She looked up and gave me a winning smile, "You know, Dr. Borysenko, your guides have been trying to contact you for quite some time. You don't listen."

I groaned inwardly, thinking of our motto, "Keep an open mind, but don't let your brain fall out." Were my boundaries so porous that I was letting in another crazy person? I winced inwardly, thinking of times when I'd done just that. But "Julie" was undaunted. "There's one guide over each of your shoulders, and they tell me you're skeptical. Right now they're showing me a scene with your face all wrapped in bandages. What a terrible accident you were in!" She ogled my face carefully. "Your nose certainly looks fine now."

I think I must have turned three shades paler at the mention of that accident from which I was still healing, physically and emotionally. It represented the nadir of a long dark night of the soul that I was still struggling to work through. As I mentioned in

Chapter 9, exhausted from work and my own unhealed fear and negativity, I had fallen asleep at the wheel of my car and caused a serious accident in 1988. Thank God the man I hit sustained only a small cut. I, on the other hand, nearly lost my nose when our Honda's shoulder harness failed, and my face hit the steering wheel.

The cosmic ticket agent went on to describe details about the accident that absolutely no one knew—not even Miron. A little chill ran up my spine, and I came promptly to attention. She lifted my luggage onto the conveyor belt and continued, "Your guides are telling me that you've been trying very hard to heal an old pattern of deep-seated fear. They want you to know that its roots are in a previous lifetime."

My eyes grew wide, and I asked rather breathily, "How do I get back to that life?"

While stapling the baggage-claim checks to my ticket jacket, she looked into my eyes. "Next time you meditate, imagine a black tunnel and tumble down it backwards." She dismissed me with a gracious smile. "Next, please."

Although I was unsure about whether I even believed in past lives, I was nonetheless very impressed by my encounter in the "twilight zone." Over the following months, I meditated and tumbled down countless tunnels backwards, but nothing in particular happened. I certainly didn't access any old memories. As I relate in *Fire in the Soul*, however, a therapist who was very skilled with past-life work soon started to stay in our home when she came in from Western Massachusetts to see clients in Boston. With her help I was able to relive very vivid scenes of a family drama that would have put *Gone with the Wind* to shame! The story was set in medieval England and involved a complex plot of betrayal, murder, and sorrow that related very specifically to the kinds of fears that had plagued me for my entire present life. After retrieving this and several other related memories, I had a series of healing dreams that culminated in the transformation of my old fears.

What really happened? I won't pretend to know whether past-life memories are literally true or not. Even Tibetan Buddhists who believe in reincarnation comment that our Western linear view of it is oversimplified. Several people who have had particularly prolonged and detailed near-death experiences believe that what appear to be past lives are in fact memories of the lives of our ancestors, all of which are stored in the genetic material within our own cells. If this is true, we have an unlimited supply of past lives to draw upon. In fact, if you do the math, it is astounding to realize that in going back only 20 generations, we each have well over a million forebears! But whether or not past-life memories are literally true, part of the collective unconscious that all people share, or the personal stories of our ancestors, their retrieval and transformation often leads to emotional healing.

Miron and I conduct an annual week-long continuing medical education course for physicians. As the doctors introduced themselves during the first session one year, a psychiatrist from the East Coast commented that she did past-life regression work. I was afraid that her revelation would shock some of the others. It did not, precisely because of her pragmatic nature. She used what worked—whether it was Prozac, dreamwork, coping skills training, standard therapy, meditation, or past-life regression. When asked whether or not she thought her clients' memories were literally true, this eclectic physician responded with a wise "I don't know." What she did know was that the "past-life" stories accessed in therapy could be uniquely healing.

This open-minded attitude is shared by another pragmatic therapist, psychiatrist Brian Weiss. His book, *Many Lives, Many Masters,* told of the therapy he did with a woman named Catherine whose phobias responded neither to medication nor talk therapy. He was trying to hypnotically regress her to the source of the traumas behind her phobias when, much to their mutual amazement, Catherine began to recount what seemed to be past lives. This was particularly unusual since neither of them had any interest in, or experience of, such things. Catherine was quite disturbed, in fact, since her Catholic upbringing certainly didn't encourage teachings on past lives! Then chairman of the Department of Psychiatry at Mt. Sinai Hospital in Miami, Dr. Weiss showed tremendous courage in publishing the account of this unusual therapy rather than sweeping it under the rug. Clearly, there is more in heaven and earth than we mortals have begun to conceive of!

Miron and I have both had a long-standing interest in a spiritual paradigm for healing. Nonetheless, encounters with psychic airport ticket agents bearing messages from spirit guides regarding the need for past-life therapy is stretching things even for me! Like my two psychiatrist colleagues, however, I am a pragmatist. Julie's message from my spirit guides did, indeed, lead to a healing when all else had failed.

So who might these spirit guides be? Some of us might think of them as guardian angels, others as the same Beings of Light who guide people through near-death experiences. Buddhists call them *devas*. Cherokees think of them as *Adawees*, the great protectors of the Four Directions. In Hebrew, the word for angel is *Malakh*, or messenger. The Iranian angel Vohu Manah (meaning Good Mind) is believed to have revealed the message of God to Zoroaster some 2,500 years ago. Similarly, the Archangel Gabriel is credited for revealing the Koran to Mohammed a thousand years later.

Although I was raised in conservative Judaism, I had no idea that Jews have a rich and living angelology, at least in our kabbalistic or mystical tradition. When my Catholic friends would pray to their guardian angels, my intellectual hackles would rise, and I would inwardly shake my head at such a silly superstition. The state of education for Jews in America was probably at its low point during my childhood and is scarcely any better today. Is there a heaven or a hell? How about a soul? Even now, you can get a group of Jews together, and they won't be able to reach a consensus on these issues. They will, however, love the debate!

It turns out that my Jewish forebears had quite a lot to say about angels. There were angels of the night and of the morning.

There were angels to protect you from evil and temptation. There were angels to help you review your life. There were the Cherubim and the Seraphim who endlessly sang God's praises— *Kadosh, Kadosh, Kadosh*: Holy, Holy, Holy is the Lord of Hosts! And there were the four great archangels: Uriel, Raphael, Michael, and Gabriel, who are invoked every night by observant Jews as they say their bedtime prayers. In fact, Jewish thought posits an almost dizzying array of angels, including the guardian angels usually associated with Catholicism!

The single best book we know about angels was written by Malcolm Godwin, entitled *Angels, an Endangered Species*. He traces the entire world history of the angels through scripture, myth, art, and modern-day therapy. Tracing the celestial hierarchy of the angels from the two foundation texts—the *Summa Theologica* of Thomas Aquinas and the *Celestial Hierarchies* of Dionysus, he delineates three triads of angels. The highest triad consists of the seraphim, cherubim, and thrones. The middle triad comprises the dominions, virtues, and powers. The lowest triad— those with whom humans knowingly interact—are the principalities, archangels, and angels. Each order of angels has a different function. The powers, for example, assist those who are lost when leaving their bodies at the time of death or who are insane. The thrones are associated with bringing the material world into manifestation from the thoughts, or word, of God.

Although Miron and I are intellectually fascinated by people's ideas about the universe, as scientists we're more impressed by data. While no one has any experimental evidence that angels exist, we do at least have what is called phenomenological evidence. Such evidence consists of first-person accounts involving angels. These reports can then be analyzed for internal consistency, such as the accounts of the near-death experience. When people of different ages, from diverse cultures, with different personal and religious beliefs, have similar experiences, science is ready to meet the angels!

A woman I'll call "Anne" shared a wonderful angel experience at one of our workshops. She was with her brother in the hospital while he was dying from AIDS. He had been very agitated until a kindly nurse arrived in his room and asked to spend time alone with him. When the nurse left an hour later, her brother was at peace. He said that he'd forgiven himself and everyone else. He was ready to go. A few hours later, her brother did pass over. But when Anne went out to the nursing station to thank the nurse who had eased her brother's transition, she was told that no one of that description had ever worked at the hospital! Many stories like Anne's can be found in the proliferation of angel books that followed Sophy Burnham's classic, *A Book of Angels*.

Near-death experiences often involve angels. The Great Being of Light who guides the soul from the body, helps the person review his or her life, and sometimes gives the person a brief tour of the Other Side is variously described as God, an angel, or something very holy. In addition, guides or masters, who are also sometimes described as angels, are a common feature of the near-death experience. In *Many Lives, Many Masters*, Brian Weiss writes of talking to these angelic guides when his patient Catherine was between lives in the Clear Light that people describe during the near-death experience. People who meet these masters in the near-death state sometimes have ongoing communication with them when they return to their bodies.

One woman we know had a near-death experience as a child. She was one of the few who got, and remembered, a rather extensive tour of the Other Side. At one point, the Great Being of Light showed her a room filled with a gray mist. In the room, there were rather depressed-looking people. By their sides were angels. When the little girl asked for an explanation, the Being of Light explained that these people were dead, but hadn't realized or accepted it. Although their guardian angels were right there, ready to help, they could not intervene because it would be a violation of free will. Help is readily available, but we must ask for it. The single most important gift this woman elicited from her near-death experience was to *remember to ask for help*.

Another near-death experiencer left his body while in the hospital, dying from complications of emergency surgery. He floated out through the door into a gray mist that was populated by some types of beings who beckoned him onwards. He followed them for a long time, what seemed like weeks in the time distortion of the out-of-body state. When he finally became concerned and challenged them to tell him who they were and where they were going, they became aggressive and began to tear him apart. Inside of himself, he heard a little voice that urged him to pray. An atheist, he knew nothing about prayer, but began to mumble things such as "God Bless America." Instantly, the aggressive beings recoiled and disappeared. Now he was alone in the mist. Again, he heard an inner voice. It was singing the old Sunday school hymn, *Jesus Loves Me*. Wondering if there really was any such being as Jesus or God, the man began to pray for help. At that moment, a Great Star of Light formed in the distance, and he sped into it. He then had a complete and loving near-death experience from which he returned a changed man.

Both of these near-death experiences, and dozens of others that we could relate, underscore *the need to ask for help*. And we don't have to wait until we're dying to do it. Some people, myself included, have a lot of trouble asking for help from anyone—angelic or mortal. My tendency is to do everything myself. That inclination, however, is slowly beginning to change because of an ancient meditation, adapted from Judaism, that I have come to rely upon. It is called The Invocation of the Angels, a practice I learned while preparing to lead a weekend spiritual retreat in the early 1990s.

Sometimes Miron and I lead retreats together, while at other times I work with a dear friend, Elizabeth (Beth) Lawrence, a former nun who married and raised four sons. We jokingly think of our work as the Jewish Mother meets Mother Superior. Beth is a pastoral counselor who is also trained in a spiritual method of healing memories called Mari-El work. This work is done with the help of the angels of the Divine Feminine. The first time we did a retreat together, a friend of ours offered the use of her large and stately home, where we spent a wonderful weekend with 50 women. The house was literally filled with angels—angel sculptures, angel paintings, and real angels whose presence was invoked by our collective prayer and intention.

We usually begin our retreats by welcoming in the Sabbath on Friday evening to sanctify our time of deep rest, spiritual communion, and celebration. In Judaism the Sabbath is thought of as a living presence, the Shekhinah, or the feminine aspect of God. The sacred space of the Sabbath is guarded by the angels of peace who are greeted with the beautiful song, *Shalom Aleichem*— "Welcome to peace, welcome to the angels of peace." One then invokes the four archangels and asks for their assistance in leading a kind, loving life. Since the first retreat that Beth and I led together in the house of the angels, these presences have continued to guide our work and to take a larger and larger part in our weekends. (You can find out more about our retreats by writing for the free *Circle of Healing* newsletter described in the Resources section of the Appendix, where you will also find information about Beth's work, through her company, The Inner Connection.)

I will describe the ritual of invoking the angels, and then, if it appeals to you, you can either record the invocation that is scripted at the end of this chapter or purchase the Hay House audiocassette, *Invocation of the Angels*, which I narrate.

The meditation is based on a Hebrew bedtime and Sabbath prayer, which translates:

> *In* the Name of God, may Michael be
> at my right, Gabriel at my left, Uriel
> before me; and above my head the
> Presence of God.[1]

This invocation, by the way, follows a very beautiful prayer of forgiveness:

> *Master* of the Universe, I hereby for-
> give anyone who angered or antago-
> nized me or who sinned against me—
> whether against my body, my property,
> my honor, or anything of mine;
> whether he did so accidentally, willful-
> ly, carelessly, or purposely; whether

---

[1]In my book, *Pocketful of Miracles*, Gabriel is invoked on the right and Michael on the left. This form of invocation was published in another source that I had drawn from previously. Since the original Hebrew prayer invokes the angels as above, we will honor that original source here.

through speech, deed, thought, or notion; whether in this transmigration or another transmigration.

The names of the four archangels are direct Hebrew translations. *El* means *of God*, and the first part of each name specifies a particular quality of God that each angel carries:

Uriel means "The light of God." The front of the body where Uriel is invoked represents the East, the place of the rising sun. The energy of Uriel concerns clarity, guidance, and new beginnings.

Michael means "The likeness of God." When I think of the Great Being of Light that people describe during the near-death experience, Michael comes to mind. Compassion, forgiveness wisdom, and love are certainly like unto God.

Raphael means "The healer of God." Physical, emotional, and spiritual healing are the aspects of God's Presence carried by Raphael.

Gabriel means "The strength of God." This angel is the emissary of the Power of the Divine Mind to create. The strength of God is love, and through Gabriel's help, we can let go of the fears and resentments that hold back the full power of our own minds to heal and create.

People sometimes make the mistake of thinking that the archangels are masculine because their names have come into common usage that way. In fact, angels are androgynous—neither male nor female—representing the Unity of Divine Mind behind all the pairs of opposites. If you could imagine the perfect union of strength and love, that would be the angelic presence that transcends gender.

Over the years I've received many letters from people who have made invoking the angels a part of their daily lives. Many of them have become used to feeling the presence of angels surrounding them, as have I. No matter what situation arises, you can always feel the safety of these divine beings protecting and supporting you. As with all forms of meditation, the formal practice prepares you for informal practice throughout the day. When I feel creatively blocked or scared, I call upon Gabriel and ask for help. If I feel grouchy and unloving, I ask for the help of Michael. When I've lost my sense of connection to a larger Whole or when I feel emotionally or physically ill, I call upon Raphael. When I need insight about something, or guidance, I ask for Uriel's assistance. I often feel the loving presence of Gabriel on my left, or the healing presence of Raphael behind me. When you feel such a presence, stop and take a letting-go breath. Listen and you may get a message.

If you remember only one thing from this book, I would hope that it might be the wonderful truth that you are never alone. From the moment that your soul became a spark in the eternal flame of Divine Being, you have been attended to by angels. Why not ask for their assistance in using the full power of your mind to heal?

INVOCATION OF THE ANGELS

Take a nice stretch and a few letting-go breaths. When you feel ready, allow your eyes to close.

Focus on your breathing, noticing the way that your whole body expands as you breathe in, and how it relaxes as you breathe out....Follow your out-breath to the point of inner stillness....

Prepare yourself to open to the angels through forgiveness. If anyone or any-thing is holding you a prisoner to resentment, you can choose to let go and be free...at least for these few min-utes. If you like, ask for Divine Help: "Great Spirit, help me forgive all those who have angered or hurt me, whether they did so willfully or care-lessly, whether through speech, thought, or action in this life or in any life. And so it is, Amen."

Now place your awareness in front of you, at the Eastern Gate of your bodily temple....Ask for the presence of the Archangel Uriel, the Light of God....Be still and notice whatever you can about Uriel's presence....Is there an area in your life where you need more clarity or guidance? Reflect on it for a minute....Now ask for Uriel's help... and know that whether in a day or a week, through a book, a friend, or a dream—help will come. Give your thanks to Uriel...and know that the presence of clarity dwells within your own soul.

Place your awareness to your right, and ask for the presence of the Archangel Michael whose name means *Like the Presence of God*....Be still and notice whatever you can about that presence....Are there any areas in your life where love or forgiveness are needed? Reflect on these situations and ask for Michael's help....Give thanks for what you will receive, and know that the presence of love and forgiveness dwells within your own soul.

Now place your awareness behind you and ask for the presence of the Archangel Raphael whose name means *The Healer of God*....Be still and notice whatever you can about the angel of healing....Do you need physical, emotional, or spiritual healing? Take a moment and reflect on whatever situations are ready for healing.... Now ask Raphael for the help you need....Give thanks to the angel of wholeness, and know that the power to heal dwells within your own soul.

Now place your awareness on your left side, and ask for the presence of the Archangel Gabriel whose name means *The Strength of God*....Be still and notice whatever you can about the power of Gabriel's creative energy. Is there any area in your own life where you require the strength of Divine Mind to overcome fear...or to bring your ideas into manifestation? Ask for Gabriel's help....Give thanks to the angel of strength, and know that strength of creative mind dwells within your own soul.

Now imagine the Great Star of Light, God's Loving Presence, over your head....Feel it raining down infinite love, mercy, healing, and forgiveness. Take in this blessing, which you have asked for by imagining it. Now take the blessing in through the top of your head and let it run through and between every cell in your body....Feel the life force....Welcome the healing....Give thanks for the Power of Love to heal.

Whenever you feel ready, come back and open your eyes, remembering that you can call upon any of the angels at any time of the day or night.

CHAPTER TWENTY-TWO

INSPIRATIONS AND AFFIRMATIONS

To Einstein, the Universe was mysterious and magnificent, awesome, and holy—a "great eternal riddle that is only partially knowable." For most of us, the riddle is posed most poignantly when our souls are on fire during stress, illness, or crisis. "Why am I sick?" "Why did this bad thing happen?" The answers we give ourselves can lead to expanded insight, connectedness, and healing, or to fear, pessimism, and isolation. Yet, even after we may have arrived at a positive viewpoint, or perhaps even a spiritual rebirth through crisis, the tendency remains to slip back into negativity—into forgetfulness of the awakenings that we have from time to time into a larger reality.

Throughout the years, I have compiled and written a number of inspirational reminders that help keep me oriented to spiritual optimism and emotional wholeness. I hope that some of these reminders will also help bring you insight, hope, and clarity when doubt and fear have temporarily clouded your vision.

It is perfectly natural to have some days when we feel hopeful and inspired and others when we feel depressed and tend to forget everything we have learned about the intrinsic goodness of life. The Greek orthodox priest Tito Colliander was once asked what monks did up there in the monastery all day long, and he replied, "We fall and get up again, fall and get up again, fall and get up again." And so it is in this greater monastery called Planet Earth.

When I co-created *On Wings of Light: Meditations for Awakening to the Source* with artist Joan Drescher, I wrote this brief cosmology about the origins of our awesome and mysterious Universe:

Once upon a time
love erupted with a mighty roar.
A ball of living, breathing light
exploded into a universe
of fire and ice, suns and moons,
plants and anmals,
you and me.
Since that first moment
love has known itself and
expanded itself through us.
Our joys and sorrows, hopes and fears,
our dissolution in night's soft womb
and re-creation in the morning's song
are reflections of the divine love
that plays its infinite melodies
on the tender strings of our hearts.
The notes of anguish, exultation and anger,
delight, pain and grace unite in a
sacred harmony when we remember that
behind all appearances,
beyond the illusion of separateness,
we are One.

In the words of the poet William Wordsworth, "Our birth is but a sleep and a forgetting, the soul that rises with us, our life's star hath elsewhere its setting." Until your star sets, may the words that follow help you to remember and to awaken from the soul's ancient sleep.

> *"That fire of clear mind is in every-*
> *one, and to remove any obscuration*
> *of its clarity is the duty of all people*
> *in this time, that each one may*
> *remember and find our way again to*
> *the source of our being."*

—Dhyani Ywahoo

"Those who are motivated by fear, no matter how they justify such motivation to themselves, are working to keep the world in darkness."

—Ken Carey

"Your pain is the breaking of the shell that encloses your understanding."

—Kahlil Gibran

"And which of you by worrying and being anxious can add one measure to his stature or to the span of his life?"

—Jesus, Matthew: 6:28

"A person who is beginning to sense the suffering of life, is, at the same time, beginning to awaken to deeper realities, truer realities. For suffering smashes to pieces the complacency of our normal fictions about reality, and forces us to become alive in a special sense—to see carefully, to feel deeply, to touch ourselves and our world in ways we have heretofore avoided. It has been said, and truly I think, that suffering is the first grace."

—Ken Wilber

"Man's main concern is not to gain pleasure or to avoid pain but rather to see a meaning in his life. That is why man is even ready to suffer, on the condition, to be sure, that his suffering has a meaning."
—Viktor Frankl

For everything there is a season
and a time for every matter under heaven:
a time to be born and a time to die
a time to plant and a time to reap
a time to break down and a time to build up
a time to weep and a time to laugh
a time to mourn and a time to dance...
a time for war and a time for peace.

—Ecclesiastes: 3

"If you realize that all things change, there is nothing you will try to hold on to. If you aren't afraid of dying, there is nothing you can't achieve."

—Lao Tzu

"Now is the only time over which we have dominion."
—Leo Tolstoy

"The present is the point where time touches eternity."
— Father Kallistos Ware

"One thing that comes out in myths is that at the bottom of the abyss comes the voice of salvation. The black moment is the moment when the real message of transformation is going to come. At the darkest moment comes the light."

—Joseph Campbell

Every situation, properly perceived, becomes an opportunity to heal.

—A Course in Miracles

"While troubles will come, they are always temporary—nothing lasts forever. Thus, there is the famous legend that King Solomon, the wisest man of all times, had a ring inscribed with the words, 'This too will pass.'"

—Rabbi Aryeh Kaplan

"Real development is not leaving things behind, as on a road, but drawing life from them, as from a root."

—G.K. Chesterton

"Somewhere in the darkest night
there always shines a small, bright light.
This light up in the heavens shines
to help our God watch over us.
When a small child is born
the light her soul does adorn.
But when our only human eyes
Look up in the lightless skies
We must always know
Even though we can't quite see
That a little light
Burns far into the night
To help our God watch over us."

—Joan Borysenko, age 10

"One of the reasons why people give
up hope is that they look at their own
contemporaries and imagine them to
be far worthier than they themselves
are."

—Rabbi Nachman

"A whole person is one who has both
walked with God and wrestled with
the devil."

—C.G. Jung

"If you deny what is your nature,
you become deeply attached to that denial.
When you accept what is there, in its truth,
then you are released.
One does not release through rejection.
One releases through love."

—Emmanuel

*"Out beyond ideas of wrongdoing and
rightdoing, there is a field. I'll meet you
there."*

—Rumi

*"God regards with merciful eyes not
what you are nor what you have been
but what you wish to be."*

—The Cloud of Unknowing

*"Bring this life into harmony with Divine purpose...
may this life come into harmony with God's Will.
May you so live that all who meet you will be uplifted,
that all who bless you will be blessed,
that all who serve you will receive the greatest satisfaction.
If any should attempt to harm you, may they contact your
thought of God and be healed."*

—Peace Pilgrim

*"Lord, make me an instrument of thy peace.
Where there is hatred, let me sow love.
Where there is injury, pardon.
Where there is doubt, faith.
Where there is despair, hope
Where there is darkness, light,
And where there is sadness, joy.*

*O, Divine Master, grant that I may not
so much seek to be consoled, as to console;
to be understood, as to understand;
to be loved, as to love;
for it is in giving that we receive,*

it is pardoning that we are pardoned,
and it is in dying that we are born to eternal life."

—St. Francis of Assissi

The Lord is my shepherd
I shall not want.
He maketh me to lie down in green pastures.
He leadeth me beside the still waters.
He restoreth my soul.
He leadeth me in paths of righteousness
For his name's sake.

Yea, though I walk through the valley
Of the Shadow of Death I fear no evil
For Thou art with me,
Thy rod and thy staff they comfort me.

Thou preparest a table before me
In the presence of mine enemies.
Thou anointest my head with oil.
My cup runneth over.
Surely goodness and mercy shall
follow me all the days of my life
And I will dwell in the house of the Lord
Forever.

—Psalm 23

"One of the basic points is kindness.
With kindness, with love and com-
passion, with this feeling that is the
essence of brotherhood, sisterhood,
one will have inner peace. This com-
passionate feeling is the basis of
inner peace."

—The Dalai Lama

"The conclusion is always the same: love is the most powerful and still the most unknown energy of the world."

—Pierre Teilhard de Chardin

"When we come to the last moment of this lifetime, and we look back across it, the only thing that's going to matter is 'what was the quality of our love?'"

—Richard Bach

"There are only two ways to live your life. One is as though nothing is a miracle. The other is as though everything is a miracle."

—Albert Einstein

The following affirmations are adapted from my book, *Pocketful of Miracles*, a daily book of spiritual practice keyed to the energies of the changing seasons.

If any of them particularly strike you, you may want to copy them onto a notecard and use them as reminders of the power of your mind to heal.

Fear is a reminder to take a deep breath and let go into the present moment where the love of the Universe is a constant support.

As I become aware of the habits of my mind, I can take a deep breath when I am spinning my gears, accessing the creativity of the present moment.

I can approach all of life like a meditation, centering in the breath, and opening to the peace that is my birthright.

I can reconnect with the inner radiance, the seed of peace and freedom in my heart, through forgiveness. As I forgive, I receive the gift of peace of mind.

I can be a radiant center of love, giving forth blessings of encouragement rather than curses of judgment and limitation.

Flexibility and the willingness to let go are helping me become more peaceful, creative, powerful, and loving.

My body feels more relaxed and comfortable as I allow myself to accept both light and shadow, becoming spacious enough to hold the paradoxes of life.

The highest vision of human life is to open my heart so that I can give and receive love.

Regardless of my outer circumstances, I know that I am completely and eternally safe.

I can respond to situations from the security of my Higher Self, letting petty irritations pass without losing my balance.

Everyone that I meet has something of importance to teach me.

I honor all relationships, particularly the difficult ones, as lessons in learning to give and receive love.

Gratitude is the natural expression of the Higher Self that brings me into the Wholeness of the moment.

I can be grateful for all situations as long as I use them as grist for the mill of soul growth.

When I remember how precious the gift of life truly is, then I feel grateful and fully alive.

Since I will reap whatever I sow, may my every action be a seed of peace and compassion—both for my own benefit and the benefit of all beings.

The awakening spirit is concerned less with perfection and more with authenticity. I am who I am.

Help is always available from the seen and the unseen worlds. It is up to me to ask for what I need, realizing that answers may come in unexpected ways.

When I put aside time for prayer, meditation and re-creation, everything flows more easily and gracefully.

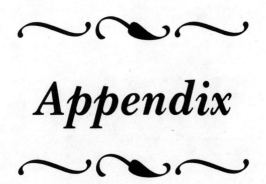

Appendix

Resources for Health and Healing

We get calls from people all over the country asking about healing programs and practitioners, types of treatment, professional training, resources, and publications. Over the years we have compiled the following list, which we hope will be helpful for you in your quest for the best healing resources. Although we have listed several healing programs, it is your responsibility to make the final decision as to whether they are right for you. We cannot recommend treatments or practitioners; we can only give you the information necessary to conduct your own investigations and make an informed choice.

HEALING-RELATED PUBLICATIONS

Circle of Healing Newsletter
Mind/Body Health Sciences, Inc.
393 Dixon Rd.
Boulder, CO 80302
(303) 440-8460
(303) 440-7580—fax

Free annual publication featuring the work of the Borysenkos, plus book reviews, articles, and a select offering of healing music, art, and meditation tapes.

Institute of Noetic Sciences
475 Gate 5 Rd.
Sausalito, CA 94965
(415) 332-5777

Quarterly Journal, Spontaneous Remission Project, issues of mind/body and consciousness. Explores the furthest reaches of what it means to be human. Excellent resource with book reviews and good mail-order catalog.

Advances
The Journal of Mind-Body Health
Subscription Dept AVN
P.O. Box 3000
Denville, NJ 07834

Quarterly journal, indispensable due to excellent abstracts of the mind/body literature from numerous journals, as well as original articles, conference reports, upcoming conferences in related areas.

Brain/Mind Bulletin
P.O. Box 42211
Los Angeles, CA 90042

Published by journalist Marilyn Ferguson, who wrote the bestselling book, *The Aquarian Conspiracy*. The Bulletin is an excellent update on research that spans mind/body medicine, physics, and consciousness.

Holistic Medicine
4101 Lake Boone Trail, Suite 201
Raleigh, NC 27607
(919) 787-5146

A quarterly journal published by the American Holistic Medicine Association. It features very readable articles on the whole gamut of complementary medicines. The American Holistic Medicine Association also has an annual conference and publishes information about that and other conferences of interest in this journal.

Common Boundary
P.O. Box 445
Mt. Morris, IL 61054
(800) 548-8737

This fine bi-monthly magazine explores the boundary between psychology and spirituality. It features a comprehensive listing of conferences and programs occurring throughout the country, many of which are continuing education opportunites in mind/body medicine and psychology.

Spindrift Inc.
Century Plaza Building
100 W. Main St, Suite 408
Lansdale, PA 19446
tel/fax (215) 361-8499

Spindrift is a not-for-profit corporation "chartered for the purpose of education and research in spiritual healing. It is an organization with a battery of repeatable tests that not only demonstrate the power of prayer, but distinguish between the effect of prayer and the placebo effect." They publish a quarterly newsletter (accompanied by an audiotape), monographs, and results of their research.

Health News and Views
Center for Advancement in Cancer Education
P.O. Box 48
Wynnewood, PA 19096-1148
(610) 642-4810

Quarterly newsletter edited by Susan Silberstein, Ph.D., who is an excellent resource person concerning conventional and complementary approaches to cancer.

International Arts-Medicine Association
3600 Market St.
Philadelphia, PA 19104

Quarterly newsletter concerning the growing field of arts-medicine.

National Wellness Association
Health Issues Update
National Wellness Institute, Inc.
1045 Clark St, Suite 210
Stevens Point, WI 54481-2962

Quarterly newsletter featuring national health care and health policy issues.

National Environmental Health Association
720 South Colorado Boulevard, Suite 970
Denver, CO 80222

Publishes the *Journal of Environmental Health* and is a clearinghouse for information on environmental illnesses. They also provide training and certification for health professionals as well as sponsoring conferences.

The Healing Healthcare Network
Kaiser and Associates
P.O. Box 339
Brighton, CO 80601
(303) 659-7995

"The Healing Healthcare Network is an association of organizations committed to developing healthcare that heals as well as cures. The Network publishes *Healing Healthcare*, maintains information resources on a variety of topics in the healing area, and operates HealthOnline, a computer bulletin board system, for individuals discussing healing and other health care topics with national leaders."

DIRECTORIES OF PRACTITIONERS
AND SUPPORT GROUPS

Holistic Health Directory
New Age Journal Publications
342 Western Avenue
Brighton, MA 02135
(617) 787-2005

This comprehensive guide lists clinics specializing in mind/body medicine, homeopathy, various kinds of bodywork, Ayurveda, massage, and a wide variety of complementary medicines. The ads are paid for by practitioners, so use your judgment wisely. As publisher David Thorne counsels, "Above all, be a responsible consumer. Many people take more care choosing a new car than they do choosing a doctor. Investigate and interview any prospective practitioner. Become a partner in your own health care. Explore all of your options." This guide has excellent tips for doing just that and certainly gives you many options for starting out, although the editors, like us, cannot endorse any specific practitioner.

The Self-Help Sourcebook
American Self-Help Clearing House
St. Clares-Riverside Medical Center
25 Pocono Rd.
Denville, NJ 07834
(201) 625-9053

This is the most complete resource for finding and forming mutual aid self-help groups.

Alternative Medicine
350 leading-edge
physicians explain their treatments.

This is an enormous sourcebook compiled by the Burton Goldberg Group to help people make informed choices from the bewildering array of available alternatives. Available from Future Medicine Publishing, Inc. (800) 641-4499

HEALING PROGRAMS

Listed below are a few of the older, more established body/mind programs. Some of them are specially designed for cancer or heart disease. The remainder are general programs for stress-related disorders and chronic illness. If you are looking for a program in your area, try calling local hospitals and universities to begin your research.

Commonweal
P.O. Box 316
Bolinas, CA 94924
(415) 868-0971

Excellent week-long retreats for cancer patients and their support persons that were featured in the Bill Moyers *Healing and the Mind* TV specials. Their director, Michael Lerner, meticulously researched and published an excellent review of complementary methods of cancer treatment called *Choices in Healing*, 1994, M.I.T. Press. Commonweal also offers very fine weekend training programs for physicians under the aegis of Rachel Naomi Remen, M.D., and staff.

ECap (Exceptional Cancer Patients)
300 Plaza Middlesex
Middletown, CT 06457
(800) 700-8869

Founded by Dr. Bernie Siegel in 1978. Offers information, support, and resources nationally. Also provides a training program for health-care professionals who wish to begin cancer support groups.

David Spiegel, M.D.
Stanford University School of Medicine
Psychiatry and Behavioral Sciences
Stanford, CA 94305
(415) 723-6421

Dr. Spiegel's support groups for women with breast cancer were featured on Bill Moyer's TV series, *Healing and the Mind.* This clinic also offers general stress management programs.

Colorado Outward Bound School
945 Pennsylvania St.
Denver, CO 80203-3198
(303) 831-6956

Offers three-day therapeutic wilderness adventures for cancer patients and their support persons.

Dean Ornish, M.D.
Preventive Medicine Institute
900 Bridgeway, Suite 2
Sausalito, CA 94965
(415) 332-2525

Dr. Ornish's studies have proven that coronary artery disease is actually reversible on a program including a no-fat-added vegetarian diet, meditation, moderate exercise, stress reduction, and social support. His institute offers week-long programs for patients under excellent medical supervision. There may also be training opportunities for professionals.

Jon Kabat-Zinn, Ph.D.
Stress Reduction and Relaxation Program
University of Massachusetts Medical Center
55 Lake Avenue North
Worcester, MA 01655
(508) 856-1616

Dr. Kabat-Zinn's ten-week mind/body program was featured on Bil Moyer's *Healing and the Mind* TV series. Some internships are usually available in his program, and many satellite programs based on his approach are springing up around the country. Call their number for regional resources. The heart of the program is described in his bestselling book, *Full Catastrophe Living*.

Herbert Benson, M.D.
Mind/Body Medical Institute
New England Deaconess Hospital
110 Francis St., Suite 1A
Boston, MA 02215
(617) 632-9525

Benson's group offers a variety of mind/body programs, some of which have been franchised by hospitals across the country. They also give a week-long training course annually through the Harvard Medical School Division of Continuing Education. Satellite programs in other cities include the following three venues:

Behavioral Medicine
Mercy Hospital and Medical Center
Stevenson Expressway at King Drive
Chicago, IL 60662
(312) 567-2259

Mind/Body Medical Institute
Morristown Memorial Hospital
95 Mt. Kemble Avenue
Morristown, NJ 07962
(201) 971-4575

Mind/Body Medical Institute
Memorial Health Care Systems
7500 Beechnut St., Suite 321
Houston, TX 77074
(713) 776-5020

Deepak Chopra, M.D.
Center for Human Potential and Mind-Body Medicine
973 B Lomas Santa Fe Dr.
Solana Beach, CA 92075
(619) 794-2425

Dr. Chopra's group provides both inpatient (week-long programs) and outpatient treatment based on mind/body approaches and on Ayurvedic medicine. This group offers seminars and trainings both to health professionals and the general public.

Ariel Kerman, Ph.D.
The HART program
645 N. Michigan Avenue, Suite 800
Chicago, IL 60611
(312) 493-4278

The HART program is a biobehavioral approach to normalize blood pressure and become medication-free when possible.

The Hoffman Institute
14 Scenic Ave
San Anselmo, CA 94960
(510) 654-2448

Miron, my son Justin, and I all went through this week-long residential program for healing the wounds of childhood, transforming old patterns, and moving into a place of compassion and forgiveness for one's parents. Individually, and as a family, it was a very important aspect of our emotional healing and spiritual growth. Based on a unique psychospiritual model, the process is affirming, yet thorough, conducted by a loving staff.

INFORMATION ABOUT SERVICES AVAILABLE

American Holistic Health Association
P.O. Box 17400
Anaheim, CA
(714) 779-6152

This educational, nonprofit association offers free literature and lists of resources for healing.

Hospicelink

A directory of hospice services in the USA and Canada, information about hospice care, and telephone support (no medical advice).
(800) 331-1620

**Office of Disease Prevention and
Health Promotion Information Center**
P.O. Box 1133
Washington, DC 20013-1133
(800) 336-4167

This office has information concerning a national project called HEALTHY PEOPLE 2000, which is supposed to be a prevention agenda for a healthy nation. Do you think they will take on the special interests such as tobacco, beef, and agribusiness whose use of organochlorine-based pesticides is likely to be one of the major causes of the increase in breast cancer from 1 in 20 women (largely postmenopausal) in 1960, to 1 in 8 women (many premenopausal) in 1993? Unless we write, lobby, and get more politically active, prevention is likely to remain in the ballpark reserved for eating Special K and getting mammograms.

Office of Alternative Medicine
National Institutes of Health, Building 31
Rm B1-C35
9000 Rockville PIke
Bethesda, MD 20892
(800) 377-4865

Established in 1992, this fledgling office is just beginning to fund research in alternative medicine sponsored by "credentialed" researchers. The first wave of thirty $30,000 grants was awarded in October, 1993.

National Cancer Institute
24-hour hotline that refers you to the cancer
information service in your area
(800) 4-CANCER

National AIDS Network
2033 M St NW, Suite 800
Washington, DC 20036
(202) 293-2437
or, for general information call (800) 342-2437

The Names Project (AIDS QUILT)
(800) USA NAME or (800) 872-6263

Children with AIDS Project of America
4020 N 20th St. Suite 101
Phoenix, AZ 85016
(602) 265-4859, HOTLINE (602) 843-8654

Children's Hospice International
901 N Washington St., Suite 700
Alexandria, VA 22314
(800) 2-4-CHILD

Ronald McDonald House Headquarters
Housing for children and parents who are away from their homes
during medical treatment.
(212) 876-1590

Alzheimer's Disease Information
(800) 621-0379

DEGREE AND CERTIFICATE PROGRAMS

We get a large number of inquiries about training in the fields of mind/body medicine and transpersonal psychology. It's difficult to provide guidance because there are so many varied routes to take. Medicine, nursing, psychology, bodywork, energy healing, and sacred music programs demonstrate some of the different approaches available. We cannot endorse particular programs. The responsibility for researching programs, their credentialing, and job opportunities post-graduation is your own.

General Points to Consider

A master's in social work (MSW) is frequently an excellent degree. It is often, though not always, insurance-reimbursable. The MSW is a two-year commitment rather than four for a Ph.D. or Psy.D., and there are often more interesting older students in such programs.

A master's in psychology may or may not lead to licensing in your state. *Research this before you begin a program* if licensure and insurance reimbursement are important for you.

Traditional Ph.D. and Psy.D. (Doctor of Psychology) programs differ in that the latter place less emphasis on research methodology and more on practical training in therapy. Both lead to insurance reimbursability and may be APA (American Psychological Association) approved. The APA, like the American Medical Association, tries to keep a tight line on professional training. In recent years, a National Register of Psychologists has appeared in which only graduates from APA-approved programs can be listed. As health-care cost containment progresses, this practice is likely to have ramifications in terms of getting insurance reimbursement.

Health psychology doctorate programs. A trip to your local library will provide you with a listing of such programs. Some are oriented toward physiological research, others to clinical practice. Finding the right program is a research project in itself. Albert Einstein Medical College in New York, the University of Rochester Medical School in New York, and the University of Southern Florida all have interesting programs.

Pastoral counseling and hospital chaplaincy programs. You can research these by calling local colleges and divinity schools.

Nursing schools. Both at the undergraduate and graduate levels nursing training has always been concerned with the whole person. More opportunities are opening for clinical nurse specialists in areas such as cardiac rehabilitation, pain management, stress reduction, non-pharmacologic control of hypertension, and other areas of mind/body medicine.

Medical schools. University of Rochester, McMaster in Canada, and Univerisity of New Mexico in Albuquerque have interesting programs that integrate at least some principles of mind/body medicine.

Bodywork, energywork, acupuncture, and Oriental healing arts are yet another avenue.

The Common Boundary Graduate Education Guide: Holistic Programs and Resources Integrating Spirituality and Psychology is a definitive guide to graduate education that will be of maximal benefit in your search.

This incredible guide is a tremendous gift and resource, written and edited by Charles Simpkinson, Douglas Wengell, and Mary Jane Casavant. It gives detailed profiles of degree and non-degree programs in psychotherapy, alternative medicine, somatic therapies, spiritual counseling, and expressive and creative arts therapies. It also contains an extensive resource list, including retreat centers, international opportunities, relevant publications, and associations.

Common Boundary, Dept. GEG
5272 River Road, Suite 650
Bethesda, MD 20816

($19.95, plus $3.50 shipping and handling)

A SAMPLING OF INNOVATIVE PROGRAMS

Naropa Institute
2130 Arapahoe Avenue
Boulder, CO 80302
(303) 546-3578

This venerable institution offers both undergraduate and some graduate degrees in Buddhist studies, bodywork, dance/movement therapy, writing, and transpersonal psychology, including Jungian psychology, music, and art therapy. They also have a wonderful summer program offering week-long and month-long continuing education opportunities. We can attest to the fact that Boulder is a great place to visit in the summer!

Rudolf Steiner Institute
Planetarium Station
P.O. Box 0990
New York, NY 10024-0541
(212) 362-2624

Rudolf Steiner was a physician who developed a spiritual science known as anthroposophy. The Institute offers college-level courses in Waldorf School education (Waldorf schools are a quickly expanding educational alternative based on spiritual values and a fine curriculum in art, music, and traditional subjects nurturing the creative impulse within each child). The Institute also offers courses in other aspects of Steiner's work.

John F. Kennedy University
Graduate School for Holistic Studies
360 Camino Pablo
Orinda, CA 94563
(510) 254-0105

J.F.K. offers master's programs in holistic health education, transpersonal psychology, arts and consciousness, and counseling psychology.

University of Santa Monica
2107 Wilshire Boulevard
Santa Monica, CA 90403
(310) 829-7402

Offers master's programs with an emphasis in spiritual psychology and certificates of completion for individuals who are not seeking degrees.

California Institute of Integral Studies
Box CB
765 Ashbury St.
San Francisco, CA 94117
(415) 753-6100

Offers both master's and doctoral programs that integrate Western and non-Western approaches to the human body, healing, and spirituality. Their somatics psychology program is a very innovative, integrative approach to bodywork.

Institute of Transpersonal Psychology
744 San Antonio Rd.
Palo Alto, CA 94303
(415) 493-4430

ITP offers both on-campus master's and doctoral programs as well as external programs involving home study and two- to seven-day intensives at various regional sites across the country. Their programs integrate traditional psychology with spiritual studies and creative expression.

CLINICAL CONTINUING EDUCATION OPPORTUNITIES

This is a very small listing of available programs offered by the clinics previously listed.

- Harvard Medical School, Deptartment of Continuing Education, under the auspices of Herbert Benson, M.D.

- University of Massachusetts Medical School in Worcester, MA, under the auspices of Jon Kabat-Zinn, Ph.D.

- Commonweal Foundation in Bolinas, CA., under the auspices of Rachel Naomi Remen, M.D.

- Preventative Medicine Institute in Sausalito, CA, under the auspices of Dean Ornish, M.D.

CERTIFICATE PROGRAMS

Academy for Guided Imagery
P.O. Box 2070
Mill Valley, CA 94942
(800) 726-2070

Drs. Martin Rossman and David Bressler, both internationally known in the fields of complementary medicine and pain management, co-chair this very fine program. Participants arrive at central sites for four-day workshops at regular intervals over a two-year period.

Jin Shin Jyutsu, Inc.
8719 E. San Alberto
Scottsdale, AZ 85258
(602) 998-9331

Jin Shin Jyutsu is one of the oldest healing arts, developed in Japan before the birth of Moses. It was brought to the United States in the 1950s by Mary Burmeister and is a marvelous way to release tensions and energy blocks that are the cause of many physical symptoms. This system of energy balancing not only involves a practitioner working with a client, but also simple and effective self-help methods. Call or write for a schedule of training workshops (these are offered throughout the United States and Europe), or to find Jin Shin Jyutsu therapists in your area. We have been personally delighted and amazed at the power of this gentle art.

The Chalice of Repose Project
554 West Broadway
Missoula, MT 59806
(406) 542-2810

The Chalice of Repose is a palliative care service and training program in musical thanatology offered at St. Patrick Hospital. The mission of the project is to "lovingly serve the physical and spiritual needs of the dying with prescriptive music; educate physicians, health-care providers, and the public about the possibility of a blessed death and the gift that conscious dying can bring to the fullness of life; integrate and model these contemplative and clinical values in daily practice. The work of this project takes place through a clinical and educational program that trains music thanatologists, recovers and expands the tradition of sacred music in assisting conscious dying, promotes and publishes historical, clinical, and contemplative research into dying as part of the life cycle; and expands and transforms cultural and medical models of the death experience." The program director is Therese Schroeder-Sheker, whose luminous recording, *Rosa Mystica*, is referred to in the music resource section. The two-year music certification includes training in voice and harp.

OTHER ORGANIZATIONS OF INTEREST

The Lionheart Foundation
c/o Robin Casarjian, M.A.
P.O. Box 194
Boston, MA 02117
(617) 965-1215

The Lionheart Prison Project is dedicated to providing healing for prisoners and taking the first steps to transform prisons into "houses of healing." Robin is the author of *Forgiveness: A Bold Choice for a Peaceful Heart*, and has brought these much-needed principles of healing into the criminal justice system. Please join us in supporting her work if you can.

The Humor Potential
Loretta LaRoche, M.D. (Mirth Doctor)
15 Peter Rd.
Plymouth, MA 02360
(508) 224-2280

We have known Loretta for years. She is hands-down the funniest wisewoman we have ever met. She has offered programs to patients and staff of the Mind/Body Medical Institute in Boston and hundreds of other hospitals, schools, and businesses across the United States. Her humor helps us to see ourselves psychologically, overcome old habits, and really use the power of the mind to heal ourselves and enjoy our lives. Write or call for a free Humor Potential Catalogue, and help stop global whining!

Murals For Healing
Joan Drescher
23 Cedar St.
Hingham, MA 02043
(617) 749-6179

Joan is an artist who has published over 25 children's books, as well as co-creating *On Wings of Light: Meditations for Awakening to the Source,* with me. Her company provides both original murals and reproductions of her murals to hospitals and clinics seeking to create a healing environment. Write or call for a free brochure.

Nightingale-Conant Corp.
7300 North Lehigh Ave.
Niles, IL 60714
(800) 525-9000

One of the leading publishers of personal development audiocassette programs. Call for your free catalog.

The Inner Connection
Elizabeth Lawrence, M.A.
P.O. Box 169
North Scituate, MA 02060
(617) 829-4303

Beth and I give four annual women's weekend spiritual retreats together. In addition, she does retreat work with other leaders, sponsors spiritual getaways to sacred sites, practices Mari-El healing—a psychospiritual mode of healing memories—and teaches laying on of hands. Write or call for a free brochure.

RECOMMENDED READING

We could write another book to encompass the book section, but we're going to show some restraint. We've foregone specific mention of some of the more popular titles such as those of Louise Hay, Dr. Bernie Siegel, Dr. Deepak Chopra, and Marianne Williamson that many of you may be familiar with, to highlight books that are lesser known or those that we've specifically referenced in the text.

Books of General Interest

The Relaxation Response. Herbert Benson and Miriam Z. Klipper. Avon Books, 1976. (The classic research findings on meditation and engaging facts about the practice of meditation in different cultures, both secular and nonsecular.)

Full Catastrophe Living: The Relaxation and Stress Reduction Program of the University of Massachusetts Medical Center. Jon Kabat-Zinn. Delacorte Press, 1990. (An excellent program of mindfulness, meditation, and healing.)

Dr. Ornish's Program for Reversing Coronary Artery Disease. Dean Ornish. Random House, 1990. (This is the only program that has been proven to actually reverse coronary artery disease.)

Natural Health, Natural Medicine: A Comprehensive Manual for Wellness and Self-Care. Andrew Weil. Houghton Mifflin, 1990.

Choices in Healing: Integrating the Best of Conventional and Complementary Approaches to Cancer. Michael Lerner. M.I.T. Press, 1994. (If you or a loved one got cancer and could get only one resource book to accompany you through the choices available for healing, this ought to be the book.)

The Healer Within: The New Medicine of Mind and Body. Steven Locke and Douglas Colligan. E.P. Dutton, 1986. (This layman's guide to research in psychoneuroimmunology is still excellent and well worth reading despite the time that has elapsed since publication.)

Healing and the Mind. Bill Moyers. Doubleday, 1993. (An excellent recap of the popular PBS series of the same title, including interviews with the healers whose clinics were featured.)

The Healing Path: A Soul Approach to Illness. Mark Barasch. Putnam Books, 1993. (An elegant first-person account of the author's healing from cancer.

Mark was at one time the editor of *New Age Journal* and had considerable wisdom and expertise to bring to his experience.)

Meaning and Medicine: A Doctor's Tales of Breakthrough and Healing. Larry Dossey. Bantam Books, 1991. (A wonderful consideration of the stories we tell ourselves that can lead to illness or healing.)

Man's Search for Meaning. Viktor Frankl. Pocket Books, 1959.
(A short, powerful book about Frankl's experiences during the holocaust and the importance of finding meaning in the midst of life's suffering.)

Healing Words: The Power of Prayer and the Practice of Medicine. Larry Dossey. Harper-Collins, 1993. (All the research ever done on prayer. Scholarly, yet very engaging.)

Recovering the Soul: A Scientific and Spiritual Search. Larry Dossey. Bantam Books, 1990. (The best overall approach to science and the spirit that we know. Highly recommended.)

The Healing Light: The Art and Method of Spiritual Healing. Agnes Sanford. Macalester Park Publishing Co., 1947. (This classic little book is still readily available and teaches everything you need to know about what Sanford calls "scientific prayer.")

The Light Beyond. Raymond Moody. Bantam, 1988. (A readable, anecdotal book that is one of the classics in near-death experience reading.)

Transformed by the Light. Melvin Morse with Paul Perry. Villard Books, 1992. (Excellent clinical case histories, first-person accounts and speculation on the meaning of the near-death experience and other light experiences to the future of humankind.)

Embraced by the Light. Betty Eadie. Gold Leaf Press, 1993. (A moving first-person account of a particularly complete and detailed near-death experience that addresses many of the questions that human beings ponder concerning the nature of the universe.)

Rituals of Healing: Using Imagery for Health and Wellness. Jeanne Achterberg, Barbara Dossey, and Leslie Kolkmeier. Bantam, 1994. (An excellent book on the use of imagery for a variety of physical complaints, and to connect with the inner-healing intelligence by three outstanding healers and researchers.)

Staying Well with Guided Imagery. Belleruth Naparsteck. Warner Books, 1994. (Belleruth is well known for her imagery audiotapes. This book contains beautiful scripts for healing imagery and an inspiring text.)

Many Lives, Many Masters. Brian Weiss, M.D. Fireside Books, 1988. (A psychiatrist's first-person account of an unorthodox but highly effective therapy involving past-life regression.)

Love Is Letting Go of Fear. Jerry Jampolsky. Celestial Arts, 1979. (A very short, pithy primer on *A Course in Miracles*, a spiritual philosophy summarized by the title of Jampolsky's book.)

The Dancing Wu Li Masters: An Overview of the New Physics. Bantam Books, 1979. (A delightfully readable book that explains the new physics and its relation to mind in a simple, exciting manner. Still topical and relevant even though it was published in 1979.)

Encounters with Qi: Exploring Chinese Medicine. David Eisenberg. Norton and Company, 1985. (Eisenberg took Bill Moyers on a tour of China. You can accompany him in this fascinating book that explores the nature of the Qi—the lifeforce energy.)

The Miracle of Mindfulness! A Manual of Meditation. Thich Nhat Hanh. Beacon Press, 1976. (A short, poetic book filled with practical advice about approaching life mindfully.)

A Gradual Awakening. Stephen Levine. Anchor Books, 1979. (Bite-size chapters on spiritual life that include excellent meditations.)

The Tibetan Book of Living and Dying. Sogyal Rinpoche. Harper San Francisco, 1992. (The classic text on Tibetan Buddhism as a practice that can enrich all spiritual paths.)

Universal Compassion. Geshe Kelsang Gyatso. Tharpa Publications, 1988. (A marvelous book on the practice of tonglen.)

Open Mind, Open Heart. Thomas Keating. Element Books, 1986. (One of my all-time favorite books on meditation.)

Forgiveness: A Bold Choice for a Peaceful Heart. Robin Casarjian. Bantam Books, 1992. (An excellent primer on one of life's most important topics.)

Appendix

Books Primarily of Professional Interest

Spontaneous Remission: An Annotated Bibliograpy. Brendan O'Regan and Caryle Hirshberg. Institute of Noetic Sciences, 1993. (This substantial text is a treasure trove for the professional who wishes to access original journal articles and abstracts that concern spontaneous remission. It is an incredible resource both for research and clinical practice.)

Psychoneuroimmunology: Second Edition. Robert Ader, David Felten, and Nicholas Cohen. Academic Press, 1991. (Edited papers of research ranging from psychoendocrinology to data on social support studies.)

The Psychobiology of Mind/Body Healing: New Concepts of Therapeutic Hypnosis. Ernest Lawrence Rossi. A Norton Professional Book, 1993. (Not for the faint of heart this highly academic, but thorough and excellent book, is a great resource for mind/body research.)

My Voice Will Go with You: The Teaching Tales of Milton H. Ericson. Sidney Rosen. Norton and Company, 1982. (The use of stories as a form of indirect hypnosis—some amazing insights here!)

The Creation of Health: Merging Traditional Medicine with Intuitive Diagnosis. Caroline Myss and C. Norman Shealy. Stillpoint Publishing, 1988. (A fine book on creating health that has a lot to say about the body's subtle energy system, including the chakras.)

Heading Toward Omega: In Search of the Meaning of the Near-Death Experience. Kenneth Ring. William Morrow and Company, 1985. (A scholarly consideration of the near-death experience that is still the best book available on the topic.)

Imagery and Disease. Jeanne Achterberg and G. Frank Lawlis. Institute for Personality and Ability Testing, 1978. (One of the classic texts for evaluating and scoring patient's imagery.)

MUSIC

Music carries us inward to the Higher Self and can provide a direct experience of the Divine. The following are some of our favorite selections for meditation, background, and ritual.

The Music of Daniel Kobialka. Daniel Kobialka is a classical violinist who composes his own music and plays the old masters beautifully, often in half-time. His tapes are particularly evocative for guided imagery and provide peaceful backgrounds for meditation. Our favorites of his many cassettes include *TImeless Motion* (the *Pachelbel Kanon* is on one side, a composition of Kobialka on the other) and *Path of Joy* (*Jesu, Joy of Man's Desiring* is on one side, a composition of Kobialka on the other).

A Feather on the Breath of God. Vocal compositions of the 12th-century Christian mystic Abbess Hildegard of Bingen. These are similar to inspired Gregorian chants and are particularly uplifting, carrying the listener inward to the Divine Silence.

Rosa Mystica, by Therese Schroeder-Sheker. Therese is a scholar of medieval music who plays the harp and sings with the voice of an angel. Rosa Mystica is an album of ancient songs about the Divine Feminine. This is one of the most beautiful, inspiring recordings we know.

Robert Gass and On Wings of Song have a series called chants from around the world. The *Allelulia*, the *Kyrie, Hara Hara, Om Namah Shivayah* and the Buddhist *Heart Sutra* on the cassette *The Heart of Perfect Wisdom* are extraordinary accompaniments for chanting or ritual. The cassettes *Ancient Mother, Many Blessings* and *Pilgrimage* are also great favorites.

Gordon Burnham is a composer and vocalist whose album, *Rhythm of Life*, we produced ourselves. His words and music are remarkably uplifting and heart-opening. As soon as we knew Gordon, we set about making his music available to the world a top priority. He also has a marvelous new album of instrumentals, produced in association with Jim Richards, called *Soul Dance*.

ABOUT THE AUTHORS

JOAN BORYSENKO, Ph.D., is the president of Mind/Body Health Sciences, Inc., and the author of the *New York Times* bestseller, *Minding the Body, Mending the Mind,* as well as *Fire in the Soul; Guilt Is the Teacher, Love Is the Lesson;* and *On Wings of Light.* She co-founded and is a former director of the Mind/Body Clinic at New England Deaconess Hospital and was an Instructor in Medicine at Harvard Medical School. One of the pioneers in the new medical synthesis called psychoneuroimmunology, Dr. Borysenko is a former cancer cell biologist, a licensed psychologist, and a yoga/meditation instructor.

MIROSLAV BORYSENKO, Ph.D., was an associate professor of anatomy and cellular biology at Tufts University School of Medicine, a former visiting professor at Harvard University, and co-founder of Mind/Body Health Sciences, Inc.

We hope you enjoyed this Hay House book.
If you would like to receive a free catalog featuring additional
Hay House books and products, or if you would like information
about the Hay Foundation, please write to:

Hay House, Inc.
P.O. Box 5100
Carlsbad, CA 92018-5100

or call:

(800) 654-5126